Acta Neurochirurgica
Supplementum 34

Peter Hindersin
Richard Heidrich
Siegfried Endler

Haemostasis in Cerebrospinal Fluid

Basic Concept of Antifibrinolytic Therapy of Subarachnoid Haemorrhage

Springer-Verlag Wien GmbH

Dr. sc. nat. PETER HINDERSIN
Dr. sc. med., Dr. phil. RICHARD HEIDRICH, Professor of Neurology
Dr. med. SIEGFRIED ENDLER

Clinic of Neurology and Psychiatry
(Head: Prof. Dr. Dr. R. HEIDRICH), Medical Academy of Erfurt,
German Democratic Republic

With 6 Figures

Originally published by Springer Wien NewYork in 1984

Library of Congress Cataloging in Publication Data. Hindersin, Peter, 1940— . Haemostasis in cerebrospinal fluid. (Acta neurochirurgica. Supplementum; 34) Bibliography: p. 1. Subarachnoid hemorrhage—Chemotherapy. 2. Antifibrinolytic agents. I. Heidrich, Richard. II. Endler, Siegfried, 1939— . III. Title. IV. Series. [DNLM: Antifibrinolytic Agents—therapeutic use. 2. Subarachnoid Hemorrhage—cerebrospinal fluid. 3. Subarachnoid Hemorrhage—drug therapy. W1 AC8861 no. 34/WL200H662h] RC394.H37H56. 1984. 616.8'1. 84-26690.

ISSN 0065-1419

ISBN 978-3-211-81839-8 ISBN 978-3-7091-4047-5 (eBook)
DOI 10.1007/978-3-7091-4047-5

Acknowledgement

We gratefully acknowledge the valuable technical assistance by our co-workers Elfriede Fischer, Edith Karpf, and Renate Sänger, and we should like to express our thanks to H. W. Kleifeld, Erfurt, Professor K. Schürmann, Mainz, and Professor Ch. Langmaid, Cardiff, for their active contribution to the accomplishment of this work.

Contents

List of Abbreviations Used

AFT	Antifibrinolytic treatment
AMCA	trans-4-Aminomethylcyclohexanecarboxylic acid-(1)
BBB	Blood brain barrier
CSF	Cerebrospinal fluid
EACA	ε-Aminocaproic acid
FDP	Fibrin(ogen) degradation products
i.th.	Intrathecal
PAMBA	p-Aminomethylbenzoic acid
SAH	Subarachnoid haemorrhage

1. Introduction

Almost a hundred years passed from the time of the first description of an intracranial aneurysm by Morgagni in 1761 to the year 1859, when Sir William Withey Gull arrived at the conclusion that haemorrhage in the subarachnoid space is caused by ruptured aneurysms. The introduction of lumbar puncture by Quincke 1891 and cerebral angiography by Moniz 1927 made it possible to establish the diagnosis of haemorrhage and its source.

In recent decades the problems of treatment have come into prominence, first of all because of the inadequacy of conservative methods of treatment in most of the cases, and from surgical experience and its limitations which became apparent before very long. Because of the erratic development of neurosurgery and vascular surgery, above all, since the technique of microsurgery has been used, the entire removal of the source of haemorrhage has become a possibility, even though there were still quite different views taken regarding the most convenient time for surgical intervention, apart from the prevailing local conditions[134, 143, 144, 261].

In an up-to-date plan of treatment of subarachnoid haemorrhage (SAH) conservative measures are appropriate for bridging the pre-operative period, and must be considered the only solution in those cases in which the source of haemorrhage cannot be found. As far as the effectiveness of such conservative therapy is concerned, the rate of rebleeding and the mortality provide sufficient comment.

Extensive studies on the enzyma systems for coagulation and fibrinolysis in the cerebrospinal fluid (CSF) were necessary, and these have formed the basis of the conservative antifibrinolytic therapy (AFT). This had aimed at optimizing the haemostasis and thus the wound healing after rupture of an aneurysm, and at inhibiting any hyperfibrinolysis.

The intrathecal (i.th.) administration of the antifibrinolytic agent PAMBA introduced for the first time by Heidrich, Markwardt, Endler and Hindersin[96, 97, 214] represents a new route for administration, and its therapeutic efficacy is under consideration in this supplement.

In this connection the following questions arose, in relation to the present state of our knowledge:

about the effect of a high content of intracellular thromboplastin in the case of disintegration of the cerebral grey matter, or damage to the cerebral vessel walls and meninges with regard to the liberated tissue plasminogen activator on haemostasis in the CSF;

about the influence by the normal or pathologically changed of blood brain barrier (BBB) resulting from a changed restricted diffusion, on the clotting and fibrinolysis proteins into the CSF space;

about the cause of fibrinolytically active CSF and localized fibrinolytic reactions during the phase of wound healing in the ruptured aneurysm and connective tissue;

about the influence of antifibrinolytic agents on these reactions, and

about possible complications of such treatment.

These phenomena are described in the individual chapters insofar as they are required for a better understanding of haemostasis in the CSF and of the drug therapy. First of all, however, some physiological and pathophysiological fundamentals on the selective action of the BBB function, biochemistry and CSF circulation are dealt with.

From the complete range of topics—*cf.* the monographs by Cervos-Navarro *et al.*[32], Felgenhauer[57], Gonsette[87], Heidrich[94, 95], Nerke[193], Pia *et al.*[213], Rapoport[222] and Schaltenbrand[236], only those aspects are described which seem to be essential for a better understanding of the haemostatic pathway and therapy.

According to our present knowledge the CSF is predominantly produced in the choroid plexuses and ependyma of the walls of the ventricles, and it then circulates from the inside of the ventricles into the subarachnoid space. CSF flows away through the arachnoidal villi into the venous system or it flows alongside the cranial and spinal nerves into the lymphatic system. CSF circulation chiefly depends on the extent of CSF production and the latter in its turn on the secretion pressure[193]. The CSF of the choroid plexuses reaches the sagittal sinus after approximately 5 hours, *i.e.,* at a velocity of 1 mm/minute.

Undirected fluid shifts are superimposed on this moderate circulation the cause of which might be found in variations in the respiration, pulse frequency, cardiac output and, last but not least, in changes of posture. Disturbances of CSF circulation arise from the anatomical narrows of the CSF space for the absorption of CSF into the superior sagittal sinus in dependence on venous pressure. An osmotic transfer of drugs due to hydrostatic and osmotic pressure gradients causing contrary effects on the CSF circulation, has been demonstrated in many experiments on i.th. therapy[47, 54, 78, 85, 142, 240]. No particular distribution pattern appears in the CSF space—with regard to pharmacokinetics—owing to the uniformly structured compartment system of CSF without any inner barriers. However, the comparatively different protein values and ratios between serum and CSF cannot be explained without supposing that a complex functional BBB system regulates the permeation between the blood and the CNS.

There is, however, in the BBB no absolute impermeability to certain serum proteins. In addition, permeability of the BBB varies in relation to the metabolism-based requirements of the structures protected by such a function. In the event that there is no insufficiency of the BBB, the normal physiological differences between blood and CSF are maintained by the Donnan equilibrium, a passive metabolic exchange, an active absorption and secretion, a diffusion into the adjacent tissue and the CSF drainage[47, 57, 87, 153, 222]. If there is a reduced barrier function of the BBB an increased protein permeation is entailed.

This, among other things, leads to the clotting and fibrinolytic pathways in the CSF to be considered typical in relation to the blood plasma system. These regulatory mechanisms of the BBB function are disturbed especially by intracranial haemorrhages (stimulus caused by a foreign body) on the basis of an inflammatory swelling of the astrocytes appendages on the basal membrane of the cerebral capillaries, having their effects by diffusion variations of the clotting and fibrinolytic factors in the CSF.

Haemostasis arrests haemorrhage, so that even in case of cerebral traumatic devasation there is no loss of blood due to controlled interactions of vascular reaction, thrombocytes, and plasmatic clotting factors. It is quite intelligible that there is a vital risk involved if those functional circles do not work in a well balanced manner in SAH patients. Hence, disturbances in correlation with the functional circles which are meaningful for haemostasis, and possible missing or reduced activities of the coagulation factors or more fibrinolytic activities give rise to direct or indirect localised or generalised tendencies to bleeding.

The coagulation pathways (*cf.* Fig. 2) represented in the monographs by Biggs[26], Deutsch[46], Bang *et al.*[18], and Fareed *et al.*[55] on the whole only guarantee under physiological conditions a firm fibrin clot and undisturbed wound healing[26,62,192,204,241].

The necessity for providing a haemostatic equilibrium is realized because of the fact that the intravascular fibrinolytic reaction which proceeds continuously is directed against the existing, but not manifest coagulation (*cf.* Fig. 2 and the monographs by Gaffney and Balkuv-Ulutin[79] and Markwardt[169]). The clotting and fibrinolytic inhibitors which produce an effect at various points on the haemostatic pathway, stabilize the haemostatic equilibrium in terms of other correction factors[43]. They will become effective only when the inactive clotting and fibrinolytic proteins circulating in the blood are activated and deployed, if required. The inhibitory proteins thus have the function of inactivating both the proenzyme (zymogen) activated at the wrong time in the wrong place and the correctly deployed enzyme after it has performed its biological function.

As inactive complex compounds they are intercepted and thus eliminated from the blood by the clearance function of the reticuloendothelial system.

The continuous turnover of these factors and thus the latent state of equilibrium may easily be disturbed by changed rates of the synthesis and breakdown, on the one hand, and by the release of natural activators such as tissue activators and vascular wall activators, on the other hand. Hence, this turnover is subject to changes and additional regularities due to the barrier function in the CSF space on the ruptured aneurysm forming a clot, and in the CSF.

The clinical effects are a local or, more rarely, a generalized activation of coagulation and/or fibrinolysis with all the consequences arising therefrom.

2. Definition of the Problems

The great efforts made in quantitative recording of the clotting and fibrinolytic relations in the CSF by means of selective analyses including objective data acquisition have in recent years brought about clarification of the haemostatic pathway with both a normal and a disturbed BBB function. It is the object of the present report[105] to revise the more or less accidental sporadic, and sometimes, contradictory results obtained in clinical research, and to complete them in accordance with the present state of knowledge, on a pathophysiological basis. In doing so, normal, inflammatorily changed and blood-stained CSF had been classified prospectively, and the activators, inhibitors, zymogens, active enzymes, the substrate and its degradation products from the haemostatic system, have been determined quantitatively.

We have been working on certain problems which at present are still unsolved. These include an intrinsic CNS synthesis of proteins in the subarachnoid space, the changed concentration gradients in disturbed BBB function, the immuno-chemically ascertained values of coagulation and fibrinolysis, steady state, formation of enzyme-inhibitor complexes, determination of the correlation between the haemostasis factors and the values of CSF proteins when there is a disturbance of BBB function and finally, determination of the proteins involved in coagulation and fibrinolysis already well known in the plasma, but not yet demonstrated in the CSF.

As far as the increased rate of rebleeding in SAH is concerned, among other things, a reaction which in most cases is locally fibrinolytic is being accepted as a working hypothesis. Follow-up studies of some haemostatic factors in the blood and the pathophysiological awareness regarding coagulation and fibrinolysis in CSF, described in the first chapter, create the prerequisite for recommending coagulation-promoting and antifibrinolytic therapy for SAH patients. According to the general assessment of oral and parenteral AFT with synthetic antifibrinolytics such as ε-aminocaproic acid (EACA) or trans-4-amino-methylcyclohexanecarboxylic acid-(1) (t-AMCHA), and in particular the behaviour of permeation of p-aminomethylbenzoic acid (PAMBA) was tested in cases of normal and impaired BBB function. In view of insufficient permeation into the CSF space—and this result may be anticipated in oral and parenteral administration—attempts had been made to explore new pathways in AFT by using the intrathecal route for administration.

The pharmacokinetic information obtained in animal experiments, after intrathecal instillation of PAMBA, included comparisons and assessments on half life, distribution, circulation and therapeutically possible limiting concentrations and their side effects. Furthermore, biotransformation of the PAMBA drug in CSF must be confirmed or excluded, and its diffusibility into fibrin clots must be determined by in vitro tests.

This report concludes with the therapeutic aspects obtained from the intrathecal instillation of PAMBA performed in SAH patients for the first time in our clinic. In addition we considered estimates to the analyses of the half-life and the side effects, as well as the diagnostic proof of an inhibited fibrinolytic reaction in the CSF.

The clinical relevance can, for the time being, be assessed only in a small unrepresentative group of SAH patients treated intrathecally without making comparisons, or making reference again to the extensive literature[2, 7, 220] regarding oral or parenteral AFT with the comparative assessment of these topics.

3. Material and Methods

3.1. Cerebrospinal Fluid Specimen

3.1.1. Normal CSF

This group comprises the cerebrospinal fluid which must be regarded as normal from a physiological point of view. With a protein concentration of < 0.35 g/l it shows a protein ratio specific to CSF in the cellulose acetate membrane pherogram, a normal immunoglobulin dispersion (IgA 0.2–5 mg/l, IgG 13–22 mg/l, IgM 0 mg/l) as well as a normal qualitative and quantitative cell count (< 5 M/l)[94]. The cerebrospinal fluid was withdrawn by lumbar puncture for establishing a diagnosis by exclusion in patients without organic neurological findings.

3.1.2. CSF Changed by Inflammation

Cerebrospinal fluid from patients with acute or chronic inflammatory lesions in the CNS was used as test material. In cases with a protein concentration of > 0.35 g/l this revealed a marked $\alpha_{1/2}$ and/or γ-globulin rise, a pathologic immunoglobulin pattern and the cell picture of inflammation (> 5 M/l).

3.1.3. Pathologically and Artificially Blood-Stained CSF

Pathologically blood-stained CSF with an erythrocyte count of > 0.05 T/l was examined as test material. The erythrocytes were predominantly haemolysed at the time of examination. The concentration of protein was between 0.45 and 8.0 g/l with an unchanged pathological mixed pherogram (type of serum). In 30% of all blood-stained CSF a rise of $\alpha_{1/2}$ and/or γ-globulin became discernible despite a marked rise in protein. IgG_S/IgG_{CSF} < 110[47,140], increased IgG and IgM values with a pleocytosis were likewise characteristic of these CSFs. In addition, artificially blood-stained CSF with an erythrocyte count of > 0.05 T/l has been prepared and tested.

3.1.4. CSF from Animal Experiments

The dogs used were 25 kg in weight and showed a total amount of CSF of 10 ml. An amount of 0.25 ml of suboccipital fluid was withdrawn four times from anaesthetized animals each[109]. A protein content of < 0.25 g/l and the normal pherograms were the criteria for physiologically normal function of the BBB.

3.2. Assay of the Coagulation and Fibrinolysis Proteins in CSF and/or Plasma

3.2.1. Immunodiffusion and Electroimmunoassay

Clarification of the coagulation and fibrinolysis in CSF and influencing them by treatment requires a profound knowledge of the enzymatic course of these reactions, including the use of selective methods for recording their activities and concentrations. Because of the low percentage of protein in the CSF, which is the material being tested, it is necessary to adapt the standardized methods appropriately, so that an accurate assessment can be made. On the basis of biophysical and kinetic enzyme activity measurements as well as immunologic concentration assays, it has become possible to record the changed ratios of coagulation and fibrinolysis in CSF as well as to follow and control by measurements in the treatment of such processes.

Quantitative determination is carried out by radial immunodiffusion, immunodiffusion-plates, M-Partigen Behring using the specific antiserum required. A quantitative determination can also be carried out by electroimmunoassay, according to Laurell[75, 98, 104, 132, 155].

Some of the active enzymes, zymogens, substrate as well as activators and inhibitors of the enzyme system of coagulation and fibrinolysis possibly present in CSF, can be detected quantitatively by direct or indirect methods.

Fibrinogen factor I (F I)
Prothrombin factor II (F II)
Factor VIII related antigen (F VIII R: Ag)
Fibrin stabilizing factor, subunit A and S (F XIII: A) (F XIII: S)
Plasminogen
Antithrombin III (AT III)
Alpha-2 macroglobulin (α-2 M)
Alpha-1 antitrypsin (α-1 AT)
C-1 esterase inhibitor (C-1 I)
Alpha-2 antiplasmin (α-2 AP), Alpha-2 plasmin inhibitor (α-2 PI)
Fibrin degradation products (FDP) and FDP fragment D (FDP: D)
FDP: D difference determination for recording the *in vitro* plasmin activity.

The final products of the plasmin-catalyzed fibrin and fibrinogen degradation are the FDP. They are the indicators and measure of a free fibrinolytic activity. By determination of the FDP in adequate stages of experiments there is the possibility (a) of excluding the extrahepatic biotransformation of PAMBA in CSF and (b) of making use of the temporary determination of the proteolytic fibrin and fibrinogen degradation as a criterion for making a distinction between the artificially and pathologically blood-stained CSF.

3.2.2. Thrombelastographic Measurements

By applying the thrombelastographic method according to Hartert (Thromb-Elastograph Hellige, Freiburg/Br., West Germany) blood and plasma samples can be recorded photokymographically at all phases of coagulation and fibrinolysis, using the factors such as reaction time, clot forming time and maximal amplitude for the estimation of the shear module[111, 211]. CSF samples must be adapted by adding plasma or fibrinogen substrate. (For further details Ref. 114).

3.2.3. *Coagulation Measurements*

The methods applied to determine the clotting process or individual factors in the blood have been described in more detail by Bang *et al.*[18], Biggs[26] and in other monographs[168,204,211,304].

Platelet count

Partial thromboplastin time (PTT)

One-stage prothrombin time, Quick value (TPT)

Fibrinogen concentration

Ethanol gelation test

Determination of the activity of plasma clotting factors in CSF, viz. prothrombin (F II), proaccelerin (F V), antihaemophilic globulin A and B (F VIII and F IX), Stuart-Prower factor (F X)[305].

3.2.4. *Fibrin Agar Plate Technique*

The heated fibrin agar plate technique permits a semi-quantitative recording of fibrinolysis which must be solely attributable to the fibrinolytic activity of the free plasmin[111,112,211].

3.2.5. *Fluorophotometric Measurements*

Almost every assessment of fibrinolytic activity is based on the measurement of the degradation of fibrin.

Hence, each estimate of a plasma and euglobulin lysis reaction[211,255] is based on a comparable time test relative to standard samples from clot formation to degradation. By marked tracer proteins (human fibrinogen substrates labelled with fluorescein-isothiocyanate) fibrinolytic reactions can be followed quantitatively in measurements in plasma and CSF by using microscope fluorometry[18,117,119].

3.3. *Determination of the Protein in CSF*

3.3.1. *CSF Total Protein*

The quantitative analysis is a *nephelometric* measurement of the protein precipitated[304].

3.3.2. *Ratios of the CSF Protein Fraction*

After a prior concentrating of the protein with collodion bags electrophoresis was carried out on cellulose acetate. Densitometric recording of the separated CSF protein fractions enables a quantitative evaluation to be made[304].

3.3.3. *Immunoglobulins*

Radial immunodiffusion according to Mancini (LC — Partigen Behring) was used for the determination of the immunoglobulins (IgA, IgG and IgM). The two methods (3.3.2. and 3.3.3.) made possible a sufficient separation into normal and pathological CSF, and a distinction between the immunoreactive and the transudative CSF syndrome.

3.4. Determination of the Concentration of Antifibrinolytic Agents from Test Materials

3.4.1. Chromatographic Determination of PAMBA

The ascending paper chromatographic wedge-tip technique with subsequent colorimetric quantitative evaluation has been used as a separation process[172].

3.4.2. Radiochemical Determination of EACA, AMCA and PAMBA

The radioactivity in the separate reaction mixtures was measured in the liquid scintillation counter LKB-Wallac 81000 by means of the tritiated compounds (^{3}H-EACA, ^{3}H-AMCA, ^{3}H-PAMBA) and then, corresponding to the specific activity converted by calculation into mg antifibrinolytic agent/l[118].

3.4.3. Determination of Aprotinin with a Chromogenic Substrate

The assay of Contrykal is based on inhibition of trypsin-catalyzed hydrolysis of the chromogenic substrate N^{α}-benzoyl-DL-arginine-p-nitroanilide-HCI. The amount of p-nitroaniline produced, which is determined photometrically at 405 nm[105, 118] is inversely proportional to the inhibition by Contrykal of trypsin-catalyzed hydrolysis.

3.4.4. Testing Materials

Concentrations of PAMBA were determined on

(a) CSF obtained from patients after a high oral dosage of PAMBA. Two hours before lumbar puncture the patients were given 6 g of PAMBA orally. Estimation was carried out as specified in 3.4.1.

(b) CSF and plasma obtained from laboratory animals after intrathecal injection of 10 to 30 mg of PAMBA.

The CSF and plasma removed at given intervals were concentrated according to the expected amount of PAMBA and estimated as specified in 3.4.1.[109].

(c) Test material for the determination of the in vitro diffusion of antifibrinolytic agents into fibrin clot in capillary tubes. The diffusability and the diffusion coefficients are determined by means of ^{3}H-labelled antifibrinolytic agents; they are calculated from the difference between the concentrations in the centrifuged clot and in the incubation solution.

3.5. Statistical Methods

A scatter of the analytical values is inevitable. However, they must be kept within certain control limits. Those control limits (permitted margin of errors) are defined by statistical values.

Hence, the formal spread was recorded by mean values, standard deviations and variation coefficients. This is followed by the calculation of the biologic scatter in the case of symmetrical and asymmetrical distributions for the individual test series.

Furthermore, for various test series the investigation has been carried out on the parity of the median values with the U test (Mann, Whitney, Wilcoxon), the calculation of the regression line and the determination of the analytical value scatter about this line (correlation coefficient). Significance tests (Welch test), in the test series to be compared, constitute the basis for the evaluation of the findings. The statistical data in here are confined to the p-values shown. They are fully presented in the original reference material[105] on which the supplementary volume is based.

4. Coagulation and Fibrinolysis in CSF

4.1. Clotting Enzyme Reactions in Normal, Inflammatorily Changed and Blood-Stained CSFs

Earlier, less definite global coagulation studies of CSF yielded sporadic indications both on the coagulation-promoting and on the inhibiting effect[94, 240]. In the light of our present knowledge attempts were made to detect some factors necessary for the endogenic and exogenic coagulation process[200, 287, 294]. Apart from some of the thrombelastographic results obtained which appeared to promote coagulation[101], the results obtained regarding the activities of the clotting factors remained contradictory. No difference was noted between normal, inflammatorily changed and blood-stained CSF. All the analyses referred to CSF, without more precise indications.

Up to the present time the question has been left open as to whether the altered permeation has any influence on the coagulation-active balance in CSF in cases of intact and disturbed BBB function.

The low physiological active and passive transport from the intracellular fluid space of the grey matter, and from the extracellular spaces via the functional brain CSF barrier permits permeation of tissue thromboplastin into the CSF[94, 110, 200, 294]. All other proteins active in coagulation which are formed in the liver and can only permeate the CSF through the blood stream (influx syndrome) are subject to selection by the BBB[57, 224]. The activities of the clotting factors in the CSF are limited by the distribution equilibria such as the half life, and the effects of CSF circulation and resorption.

The thrombelastographic analyses of CSF-plasma mixtures as against plasma verify a coagulation-promoting effect ($p < 0.001$), notwithstanding the fact that the proportion added might be normal, inflammatorily changed or blood-stained CSF. There are no significant differences ($p > 0.05$) between the normal and pathological CSF-plasma reaction mixtures. The activation of coagulation initiated by adding CSF to the plasma can only be

Table 1. *Analytical Values of the Coagulation Factors in CSF.* Thrombelastographic determination of the variation in the coagulation activity in plasma produced by adding CSF and 0.025 M $CaCl_2$ solution in a ratio of 1:1:1. Activity values in proportions to the coefficient factor 1 and immunochemical determination of concentrations in mg/l or percent of the normal

Methods and normal values in plasma	Normal CSF (n) ($\bar{x} \pm s$)	CSF changed by inflammation (n) ($\bar{x} \pm s$)	Pathological or artificial blood-stained CSF (n) ($\bar{x} \pm s$)
Thrombelastography	n = 15	n = 20	n = 20
r-value (s) 586 ± 166	189 ± 41	201 ± 154	174 ± 102
k-value (s) 1,335 ± 408	110 ± 43	275 ± 130	245 ± 136
Factor II	n = 35	n = 35	n = 35
concentration (mg/l) 60–100	0.9 ± 1.44	2.2 ± 2.43	9.2 ± 5.39
Factor VIII	n = 50	n = 35	n = 20
related antigen 0.47–1.85	< 0.005	< 0.005	0.021 ± 0.053
Factor XIII	n = 20	n = 20	n = 20
subunit A 0.30–1.60	< 0.010	< 0.010	< 0.010
Factor XIII	n = 20	n = 20	n = 20
subunit S 0.50–1.50	< 0.010	< 0.010	0.035 ± 0.075
Factor II activity	n = 50	n = 50	n = 50
(0.75–1.20)	0.005 ± 0.003	0.007 ± 0.003	0.072 ± 0.009
Factor V activity	n = 35	n = 35	n = 35
(0.75–1.20)	0.030 ± 0.030	0.022 ± 0.022	0.058 ± 0.039
Factor VIII activity	n = 50	n = 50	n = 50
(0.70–2.00)	0.020 ± 0.013	0.021 ± 0.010	0.022 ± 0.014
Factor IX activity	n = 50	n = 50	n = 35
(0.70–2.00)	0.023 ± 0.020	0.066 ± 0.125	0.090 ± 0.151
Factor X activity	n = 50	n = 50	n = 50
(0.75–1.20)	0.009 ± 0.010	0.007 ± 0.009	0.059 ± 0.042

produced by a concentration of thromboplastin in the CSF. It is maintained by transudative and diffusible processes between the grey matter rich in thromboplastin and the CSF[15, 107, 174, 265].

As is shown in Table 1 there is only a partial correlation between the increased permeation of the predominantly high-molecular clotting factors and any BBB disturbance as regards activity values such as F II, V, VIII, IX and X, and the concentration values such as F II, F VIII R: Ag, F XIII_A, and F XIII_S. Possible causes of the absent permeation are the high molecular weight[204,305] and the unfavourable steric molecular arrangement[58]. In addition, in case of CSF affected by inflammation the relatively slight increase in the clotting factors as compared to the raised protein values, may also be the effect of an immunoreactive process in the CNS.

Pathological or artificial blood-stained CSF differs significantly ($p < 0.001$) in its clotting activities from the inflammatorily changed and normal CSF during the process of clotting, despite the assumed consumption of factors. The demonstrated activity values are based upon the assumption that the fibrinogen substrate emerging with the blood predominantly is subject to fibrin coagulation before it becomes detectable always as FDP in the blood-stained CSF, by the subsequent fibrinolytic reaction. The increase of F XIII: A in blood-stained CSF, absent in relationship to the protein increase, also substantiates a completed coagulation reaction.

Hence, the fibrin moiety can already be decomposed into soluble FDP from the intermediarily formed fibrin deposition thrombus, by the time of examination (CSF removal), so that the visual impression of "non clotting blood" in CSF[94,240] must be revised in the light of our present-day knowledge[107].

4.2. Protein Coagulation Inhibitors in Cases of a Normal and Disturbed BBB Function

The coagulation inhibitors limit the thrombin activity no longer necessary in the blood from a physiological aspect, and maintain predominantly the balance of the coagulation[246].

Several authors[94] have detected anticoagulatory proteins by applying non-selective methods of detection while investigating some CSFs. They have postulated that in certain neurologic diseases which have not yet been more closely identified, CNS-intrinsic proteins would have a coagulation inhibiting effect. Above all, in cases of tuberculous meningitis, proteins with antithrombin-like activity are said to show a coagulation inhibiting effect.

More recent reports, published since 1961, are not contained in the relevant reference material[105].

According to our present knowledge, only the thrombin neutralizing proteins are of significance. The activities of AT I and AT VI form the minor part of the thrombin neutralizing potential, whereas AT III and α_2M exert a correlating dual function between coagulation and fibrinolysis inhibition[18,26,55,173].

The α_2M and AT III concentrations in normal and the increased values in inflammatorily changed and blood-stained CSF are dealt with as specified in the description of the fibrinolytic inhibitors. It is apparent in this connection, that the increased concentrations of α_2M and AT III have no measurable inhibitory influence on the clotting pathway after impairment of the cerebral barrier function, otherwise the fibrinogen emerging with the blood would be detectable immunochemically. However, this is not the case (Table 3).

4.3. Fibrinolytic Enzyme Reactions in Normal CSF, CSF Changed by Inflammation and Blood-Stained CSFs

It has been observed[89,94,100,223,230,255] that the fibrin and fibrinogen portions of haematomas predominantly remain fluid in serous cavities as a result of defibrination. This has given rise to the assumption that CSF almost always shows a fibrinolytic activity. In accordance with the state of knowledge at that time very detailed examination and analysis of the CSF was undertaken in patients with neurological diseases[99,101,139], after myelography[139,216,242,262], in intracranial haemorrhage[216,263] and also in experimental cerebral haemorrhage in animals[76,184,185,250]. The findings in these tests always showed an "incomplete fibrinolytic activity" or inactive plasminogen activator.

The broad scatter of the results so far obtained in the abovementioned publications is probably caused by analytical methods which are not, but predominantly by a partially pathologic protein structure. Hence, it is fundamentally necessary to differentiate between normal and pathological CSF[111].

According to the latest findings by Tovi[268,272,274] and other authors[8,59,112,114,279] a free fibrinolytic activity in the case of inflammatorily changed CSF can only be assumed, if plasma proteins penetrate the CSF. Such a permeation of protein occurs as a result of local inflammatory lesions acting on the pial vascular endothelium (transudative CSF syndrome), or by bleeding into the CSF spaces[124,268,274]. In particular, the intrinsic plasminogen activators present in the shed blood increase the amount of plasminogen activators already present in the CSF. The question raised as to the origin of the activators and their correlating rise in concentration in the case of a transudative CSF syndrome is already being investigated experimentally by a great number of authors[4,12,13,166,187,207,262,268,269]. It seemed reasonable to suppose that the extrinsic plasminogen activators (cytokinases) increasingly released especially in case of necrosis from inflamed vascular endothelium[131], as well as meningeal cells and cells of the choroid plexus, were the cause of the fibrinolytic activity[79,256].

This theory only applies to the pathogenesis of increased fibrinolysis, provided that there is sufficient concentration of plasminogen in the CSF[111,112].

As the CSF shows proteins which are specific to serum and CSF[240], and do not correspond to the ultrafiltrate of the plasma it must be established whether, in the case of an intact BBB function, proteins necessary for the enzymatic process of fibrinolysis enter the CSF or whether they are formed there locally (cerebrogenesis).

Even under physiological conditions the CSF, which is produced in the choroid plexus and the cerebral ventricles, shows an increase in protein as it flows in a caudal direction. This can only be explained by processes of diffusion, resorption and transudation on the boundary surfaces of the external CSF spaces and the ventricle walls, as well as by protein diffusion from the meningeal vessels.

According to the prevailing opinion[57,224] these are the only criteria for the physiologically mutual protein reactions between the boundary surfaces of the leptomeninx, the vascular system and CSF when considering the selective separation effect of biological membranes.

The results obtained by us, indicated in Table 2[105] show that under physiological conditions—in contrast to serum—the concentrations of F-I are more than 1,000 times, and those of plasminogen are about 100 times lower, and that there was no free plasmin activity recorded. For this reason the CSF space must be regarded as a compartment insulated to a large extent by the BBB function[47]. The high content of plasminogen activators[12,13,48,166,187,207,215,262,268] detected by several authors does not become effective in the same way as the reaction initiating protein, owing to the fact that the amounts of plasminogen have fallen far below the amount required to bring about an enzymatic fibrinolytic reaction. Normal CSF therefore cannot be regarded as a fibrinolytically active fluid[111].

From the results of an inflammatorily changed and blood-stained CSF it can also be deduced that, with an increase in the exchange processes in the meningeal boundary surfaces (transudative CSF syndrome), such increase is accompanied by a chemical protein change, which frequently results in a completion of the proteins required for fibrinolysis. Therefore the inflammatorily changed and more especially the blood-stained CSF show a more or less marked plasmin activity. Liberated plasminogen activators and plasminogen permeated with the blood, or diffused because of the existing concentration gradient when there is a disturbance of the BBB function[194, 298], facilitate a plasmin-catalyzed fibrin and fibrinogenic degradation reaction, and become manifest in immunochemically detectable amounts of FDP (FDP-D, FDP-E).

A requirement for this is the fibrin and fibrinogen that has been present, which for instance, in the case of tuberculous meningo-encephalitis is frequently not subject to any proteolysis, and thus exists as a macroscopically discernible "spider web clot". After adding streptokinase-activated plasma or human plasmin, the fibrin clots were broken down proteolytically into FDP. In cases of CSFs changed by inflammation there is no correlation between the increasing protein and FDP concentration, although these two factors often go together in the case of disturbed BBB function[30, 123]. The values show a lot of scatter because of the different turnover[148], and do not correspond to the severity of the clinical picture.

As is apparent in Table 2, the increase in the protein shows some correlation with the plasminogen concentration[194, 298]. In the case of blood-stained CSF, the fraction of the plasminogen coming in directly with the blood superimposes itself additively, so that the first requirement for a still more intense fibrinolytic reaction has been satisfied.

Disregarding the results[105, 112] just referred to, there must be other explanations, as the significantly ($p < 0.001$) increased fibrinolytic activity of blood-stained CSF[8, 49, 268, 272] must have other causes as well in relation to CSF changed by inflammation. In addition to the already existing intrinsic CSF plasminogen activators and because of the concentration increased as a result of the pathological transudative processes the blood constituents likewise produce tissue activators (erythrokinases, leucocyte activator) during the cytolysis[79, 105, 110, 112] as the second prerequisite for an increased fibrinolytic activity[105]. Furthermore, the granulocytic and endothelial content of plasminogen which is still being set free must be given due consideration in the total balance[19, 79].

The concentrations of inherent fibrinogen substrate required for the demonstration of fibrinolysis from normal and inflammatorily changed CSF and for recording an optimum fibrinolysis process, have markedly fallen or no longer exist. For this reason, it is

Table 2. *Determination of Concentrations and Activities of Fibrinolysis Factors in Normal CSF, and in CSF Changed by Inflammation and Contaminated with Blood Naturally and Artificially*

Factors, methods	Normal CSF protein value < 350 mg/l	CSF changed by inflammation protein value > 350 mg/l	Blood-stained CSF protein value ≫ 350 mg/l
Fibrinogen concentration	n = 100 100 CSF < 5 μg/ml CSF 5–10 μg/ml CSF > 10 μg/ml	n = 25 21 CSF < 5 μg/ml CSF 5–10 μg/ml 4 CSF > 10 μg/ml	n = 25 pathologically blood-stained 25 CSF < 5 μg/ml CSF 5–10 μg/ml CSF > 10 μg/ml
Plasminogen concentration	n = 100 100 CSF < 5 μg/ml CSF 5–10 μg/ml CSF > 10 μg/ml	n = 100 81 CSF < 5 μg/ml 12 CSF 5–10 μg/ml 7 CSF > 10 μg/ml	n = 25 pathologically blood-stained CSF < 5 μg/ml 14 CSF 5–10 μg/ml 11 CSF > 10 μg/ml
In vivo plasmin activity determination by FDP values	n = 100 100 CSF < 5 μg/ml CSF 5–10 μg/ml CSF > 10 μg/ml	n = 50 45 CSF < 5 μg/ml 2 CSF 5–10 μg/ml 3 CSF > 10 μg/ml	n = 25 pathologically blood-stained 2 CSF < 5 μg/ml 4 CSF 5–10 μg/ml 19 CSF > 10 μg/ml
Plasmin activity, 24-hour incubation mixture by adding plasma, determination by FDP values	n = 25 18 CSF < 5 μg/ml 4 CSF 5–10 μg/ml 3 CSF > 10 μg/ml	n = 25 17 CSF < 5 μg/ml 7 CSF 5–10 μg/ml 1 CSF > 10 μg/ml	n = 150 artificially blood-stained 26 CSF < 5 μg/ml 34 CSF 5–10 μg/ml 90 CSF > 10 μg/ml

Plasmin activity TEG mixture with plasma/CSF of a ratio of 1:2	n = 25 ($\bar{x} \pm 2s$) 25 CSF 0–21% $\bar{x}_{ma}$ = 25 mm	n = 25 13 CSF < 20% 8 CSF 20–30% 4 CSF > 30% $\bar{x}_{ma}$ = 39 mm	n = 25 artificically blood-stained 13 CSF < 20% 10 CSF 20–30% 2 CSF > 30% $\bar{x}_{ma}$ = 37 mm
Plasmin activity TEG mixture with KABI-human research fibrinogen/CSF of a ratio of 1:2	n = 25 ($\bar{x} \pm 2s$) 25 CSF 0–5% $\bar{x}_{ma}$ = 34 mm	n = 25 CSF < 5% 10 CSF 5–15% 15 CSF > 15% $\bar{x}_{ma}$ = 26 mm	n = 25 artificially blood-stained 1 CSF < 5% 16 CSF 5–15% 8 CSF > 15% $\bar{x}_{ma}$ = 29 mm
Plasmin activity heated fibrin agar plate technique	n = 50 50 CSF < 7 mm^2 lysis area	n = 50 50 CSF < 7 mm^2 lysis area	n = 50 artificially blood-stained 45 CSF < 7 mm^2 lysis area 5 CSF 7–17 mm^2 lysis area CSF > 17 mm^2 lysis area

necessary to add to the reaction mixture some extraneous fibrinogen in order to saturate the substrate and thus ensure an optimum enzyme-catalyzed reaction according to Michaelis and Menten[105,114].

With normal CSFs objective measurement is facilitated by adding only fibrinogen. In the case of CSFs changed by inflammation significant differences ($p < 0.01$) appear in the extent of the fibrinolytic activity, so that in summary the determination of plasmin catalyzed activity can always be achieved by demonstrating saturation of the F I substrate. This is verified by the immunochemical and thrombelastographic determinations[114] of the fibrinolytic CSF activity (Table 2).

4.4. Proteins Which Inhibit Fibrinolysis in Cases of Normal and Disturbed BBB Function

The axiom "action and reaction are equal and opposite" holds true in the blood for the coagulation and fibrinolytic pathways and for the assessment of the fibrinolysis ratio, but it must still be cleared up whether this also applies to the CSF.

In the blood the fibrinolytic active plasmin is faced with a great number of protein inhibitors which are capable of inhibiting the fibrinolytic reaction to a certain stage both as regards time and also extent. The inhibitors directed in their enzyme specificity predominantly to plasmin are the progressively acting α_1 antitrypsin, antithrombin III and the C-1 inactivator, as well as the immediately acting α-2 antiplasmin (fast-acting plasmin inhibitor)[173,178] and α-2 macroglobulin. Such an inhibitor protective function in the plasma in comparison to the active enzyme plasmin is designed in such a way that fibrinolytic enzyme reactions can be fully compensated[79]. Only when the reaction rate between the inhibitor and active enzyme does not suffice to bind all the plasmin molecules immediately, there is the possibility of another reaction with the substrate fibrin or fibrinogen[79]. A measurable fibrinolytic activity can result from this.

There is evidence of some intact and some disturbed BBB functions in considering the following results and the extent to which these inhibitors will become effective and their presence in the CSF is substantiated[115].

α-1 antitrypsin and α-2 macroglobulin were detected as trace proteins[243] in sporadic examinations of various CSFs. The regularity of the present "restricted diffusion"[57] in the case of normal CSF, also led one to expect an antithrombin III and C-1 inactivator concentration which could readily be determined immunochemically as to its quantity[115].

If pathologically increased protein permeation is present in the case of inflammatory reactions in the CNS, the influence of the BBB selection on the quantity of the inhibitor ratio must be regarded as decisive. When active protein transfer and cerebrogenesis are absent it can be gathered from Table 3 that, when the protein value increases, the inhibitors will not increase to the same extent. The selection of the passive protein transfer in the glial zones is predominantly dependent on the relative molecular weight, the steric arrangement and hydrodynamic volume of the inhibitors[47, 57, 58]. This is apparent from the results as indicated in Table 3. In the case of CSF changed by inflammation the usually dominating selective separation effect for the molecules of proteins recedes[47]. The low molecular weight proteins antithrombin III, α-2 antiplasmin and α-1 antitrypsin may now increasingly enter the CSF in contrast to the α-2 macroglobulin with high molecular weight whose values remain almost constant[140]. For that reason, slightly increased α-1 antitrypsin and antithrombin III values are a very sensitive indicator of disturbances of the BBB function (influx syndrome). In cases of haemorrhages with a direct inflow of blood into the CSF space there will be changes in relationship to the amount of blood which enters and the effect of dilution by CSF and fluid turnover. Hence, pathologically changed diffusion, absorption and transudation processes will be produced, and due to the biological elimination half-life, the result will be slightly changed protein patterns in response to the composition of plasma[115].

At present, no diagnostic importance should be attached to the determination of the plasmin inhibitors in the CSF. Statements cannot be made in an individual case, disregarding the detection of a disturbance in the steady state equilibrium.

In all reversible reaction paths, leading to a free plasmin phase, the still absent interaction between the enzyme and inhibitors must be taken into consideration[112, 255, 268, 296]. The latter is produced by the entirely low concentration of inhibitors, and is intensified even more by the dilution effect of CSF. A dissociation of the stable, biologically inactive inhibitor-enzyme complex under high inhibitor concentrations in the plasma[79, 257, 295, 296] explains the findings related to the fibrinolytically active CSF in the group of bleedings and in cases of inflammatory reactions in the CNS[105, 112, 114, 268].

To summarize it must be stated at the end of this chapter that up

Table 3. *Physiological Inhibitors of Fibrinolysis in Normal CSF, in CSF Changed by Inflammation and Blood-stained CSF.* Italic figures: The inhibitor values have been converted, in compliance with the ratio, to the CSF protein levels

Physiological inhibitors	Molecular weight (daltons)	Interaction between Plasmin = P Thrombin = T Kallikrein = K P	 T	 K	Concentration in plasma or serum (70 g/l) (mg/l)	Concentration in CSF from the "Literature" (mg/l)	Normal CSF protein value $\bar{x} = 240$ (mg/l)	CSF changed by inflammation protein value $\bar{x} = 706$ (mg/l)	Pathologically blood-stained CSF protein value $\bar{x} = 2,470$ (mg/l)
α-2 macro-globulin (α-2 M)	800,000	+	+	+	2,600 ± 700 (3.3 μmol)	1–5	n = 121 *9.0* $\bar{x} = 2.5$	n = 63 *26.2* $\bar{x} = 2.9$	n = 20 *91.7* $\bar{x} = 13.2$
α-2 plasmin inhibitor (α-2 PI, α-2 AP)	65,000	+	+	+	60 ± 10 (0.95 μmol)	0.2–0.3	n = 40 *0.2* $\bar{x} = <0.2$	n = 20 *0.6* $\bar{x} = <0.2$	n = 20 *2.1* $\bar{x} = <1.0$
α-1 anti-trypsin (α-1 AT)	54,000	+	—	+	2,900 ± 450 (54.0 μmol)	5–16	n = 121 *10.0* $\bar{x} = 5.9$	n = 63 *29.4* $\bar{x} = 10.7$	n = 20 *102.3* $\bar{x} = 35.1$
Antithrombin III (AT III)	65,000	+	+	—	290 ± 29 (4.5 μmol)	no indications from literature	n = 121 *1.0* $\bar{x} = 2.4$	n = 63 *2.9* $\bar{x} = 4.2$	n = 20 *10.2* $\bar{x} = 8.0$
C-1 esterase inhibitor (C-1 I)	104,000	+	—	+	230 ± 30 (2.3 μmol)	no indications from literature	n = 121 *0.8* $\bar{x} = 0.1$	n = 63 *2.3* $\bar{x} = 1.9$	n = 20 *8.1* $\bar{x} = 6.0$

to some years ago fibrinolytic reactions in the CSF could only be suspected or else diagnosed by their effects. Irrespective of the fact if the present studies had been performed with or without substrate saturation, they are appropriate to differential diagnosis. Only in this way is it possible for the clinician to make a therapeutically effective intervention in certain cases.

4.5. Technique for Differentiating Between Artificially and Pathologically Blood-Stained CSF

In the case of a bloody CSF, a distinction must be made whether it is an intrinsically blood-stained CSF, or whether the blood admixture originates iatrogenically from a lesion of a spinal vessel at the time of the diagnostic lumbar puncture[94, 223, 229, 240]. In spite of several possibilities of differentiation such as xanthochromia, assessment of the qualitative and quantitative CSF cell picture, determination of oxyhaemoglobin and the benzidine reaction as well as the detection of visible formation of streaks and clot when the CSF-blood mixture extravasates[94, 240, 281], there is often uncertainty about the assessment of a blood-stained CSF.

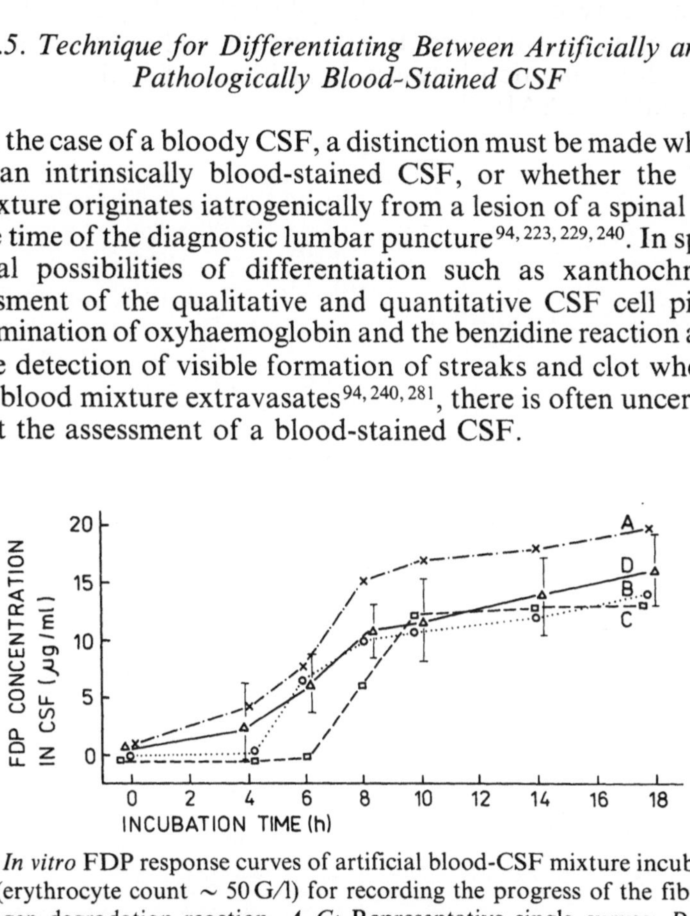

Fig. 1. *In vitro* FDP response curves of artificial blood-CSF mixture incubated at 37 °C (erythrocyte count ~ 50 G/l) for recording the progress of the fibrin and fibrinogen degradation reaction. *A–C:* Representative single curves: *D:* Mean value curves at n = 30 and ($\bar{x} \pm 2\,s$)

Another possibility of differentiating an artificially blood-stained CSF is that the fibrin and fibrinogen degradation reaction has not yet started (negative FDP detection, < 5 µg/ml), in contrast to the pathologically blood-stained CSF that must at all times be regarded as fibrinolytically active (positive FDP detection, $\gg 5\,\mu g/ml$)[113]. FDP determinations in the CSF can be performed quite easily, and may complete the diagnostic spectrum.

According to the reaction-time curves as plotted in Fig. 1, a positive detection of FDP in the blood-stained CSF must result, not only five hours after artificially adding blood, but even six hours after the entry of blood into the subarachnoid space. The time interval of up to five hours after the withdrawal of CSF, permits a definite differentiation between an artificially blood-stained CSF and an intrinsic SAH[113].

5. Sequence of Haemostasis in SAH

5.1. Risk of a Recurrent SAH

A subarachnoid haemorrhage is caused in 60 to 70% of all cases by a ruptured saccular aneurysm or an arteriovenous malformation, due to a faulty vessel wall and temporary rises in blood pressure[25, 51, 78, 94, 95, 146, 288].

The prognosis is directly dependent on the severity of the bleeding in the subarachnoid space, on the extent of the cerebral injury and the effects on the cerebral metabolism, on the liberation of the vasoneuroactive substances such as bradykinin, on the development of oedema and on the number and timing of rebleeding. In addition to the regional cerebral blood flow (rCBF) and the level of the intracranial pressure, the vasoactive, coagulation and fibrinolytic reactions in terms of risk factors should be observed. The latter may promote or delay the natural occlusion of the rupture aneurysm by haemostatic plug formation and subsequent consolidation[61, 165, 201, 233, 238].

5.2. Cerebral Vasospasm as a Factor Influencing Aneurysmal Bleeding

The urgent formation of a thrombus on the fundus of a ruptured aneurysm without any delay is also dependent on the regulation of the lumen of the neighbouring vessel and the blocking-off mechanism of the vascular lesion. Among the vascular reactions ensuring partial occlusion, distal and proximal to the ruptured aneurysm, it is an immediate neurogenic, adrenergic vasoconstriction due to the lesion of the vessel wall and a slightly passive vasoretraction due to the pressure drop in the vessel, that must be differentiated from a later vasoconstriction due to vasoactive substances[39, 55, 90, 186, 213, 248]. The severity of haemorrhage and the prognosis are strongly influenced by these reactions. A delayed or slight vasoconstriction at the onset of bleeding has the effect of an intensified extravasation up to the arrest of the bleeding by the intermediary platelet plug. Vasoconstriction becomes effective in the different parts of the vessel partly with small portions of vascular smooth muscle cells

Table 4. *The Most Important Vasoactive Agents Which Constrict Cerebral Blood Vessels (A), Blood and Other Constituents of a Similar Effect (B), and Factors Which Exacerbate Vasospasm by Causing Vasoconstrictor Supersensitivity of Cerebral Blood Vessels (C)*

Serotonin and its metabolites	(A and B)
Catecholamines: Adrenalin and noradrenalin;	(C)
with involvement of sympathetic nervous system	(A and C)
Histamine	(A and B)
Angiotensin and other neuropeptides	(A and B)
Prostaglandins ($PGF_{2\alpha}$) and thromboxane-A_2 (TxA_2)	(A and B)
Vasopressin	(A)
Erythrocyte breakdown products, oxyhaemoglobin, whole blood	(B)
Fibrin/fibrinogen degradation products, FDP-D, FDP-E and fibrinopeptides A and B	(B)
Thrombin	(B)
Blood constituents, partially haemolysed, increased K^+ion concentration in CSF	(C)
Vasoconstrictor factor(s) in haemorrhagic CSF (circulating immune complexes)	(C)
Reduced production of the vasodilator prostacyclin	(A indirect)

and in the case of arteriosclerotically changed cerebral vessels to a varying degree[32,192,213]. Vasoactive substances, which not only increase the sensitivity of the vessels to vasoconstriction but also act as vasoconstrictors, emerge during the commencing platelet adhesion, the formation of the haemostatic platelet plug, right up to the phase of proliferation of the wound healing. They are listed here with acknowledgement to the Tables by Towart[3,162,276].

With morphologically intact vessels an increased resistance to flow is produced by the biochemically released cerebral vasospasm on both sides of the ruptured aneurysm, linked with an increase in the rate of arterial blood flow[110,182]. The various forms of aneurysm also set up in the immediate surroundings varied and intense turbulence in the blood flow that is usually laminar[94,182,227]. This turbulence has a negative effect on the haemostasis mechanism[110].

A raised blood pressure is likewise held jointly responsible for the degree of severity of a SAH and the risk of rebleeding[94,95,213]. A return to normal haemodynamics, should therefore be the aim of treatment.

The reduced rCBF of the brain due to the rise of intracranial pressure together with oedema formation[22,81] is favourable to the mechanisms of haemostasis, but in the case of a vascular system previously damaged by arteriosclerosis it contributes particularly to the deterioration in the general ischaemic situation[54, 64, 90, 157]. An acidosis around the basilar arteries occurring incidentally after SAH promotes the formation of thromboxane-A_2[260]. The hypoxia frequently co-existing with vasospasm must be held responsible also for biochemical damage to the vascular walls in the brain[18, 151], which causes a release of the vascular wall plasminogen activator[150].

Since the duration of the first active vasoconstriction distal and proximal to the aneurysm rupture is transitory[213], it is the coagulation mechanisms leading to the rapid formation of the platelet plug and later to the formation of the depositing thrombus which are decisive for a rapid occlusion of the rupture. The particularly intensive vasospasm, which occurs three to four days after an SAH, and has an unfavourable effect on the haemostasis, is according to Towart predominantly due to the Ca^{++}-induced activation of the contractile elements[213, 276]. The possibility of an influx of free calcium into the vascular smooth muscle cells may be inhibited by selective calcium antagonists[266, 276]. Other promising measures for the prevention of cerebral vasospasm after SAH[61] have included the application of sodium nitrite (10 mM) solution to the surface of the arteries during operation[206, 213] and the use of thromboxane synthetase inhibitors or $NaHCO_3$[235, 259]. The good results discernible on a CT scan obtained by administering these drugs, have decisively changed the prognosis and the timing of operation. Likewise early operation and washout of blood clots (extensive clot evacuation) should be suitable for the prevention of cerebral vasospasm[205, 209].

5.3. Coagulation Reactions and Thrombus Formation After Bleeding from an Aneurysm

Every aneurysmal rupture, in the course of which the blood entering the subarachnoid space, comes into contact with the intrinsic thromboplastic factors from the vessel wall, sets off a process of coagulation[26, 42, 55, 154, 192, 204].

Because of the tissue thromboplastin set free from the damaged vessel wall, the path via the extrinsic clotting system is for the time being of paramount importance for the sealing of the source of bleeding.

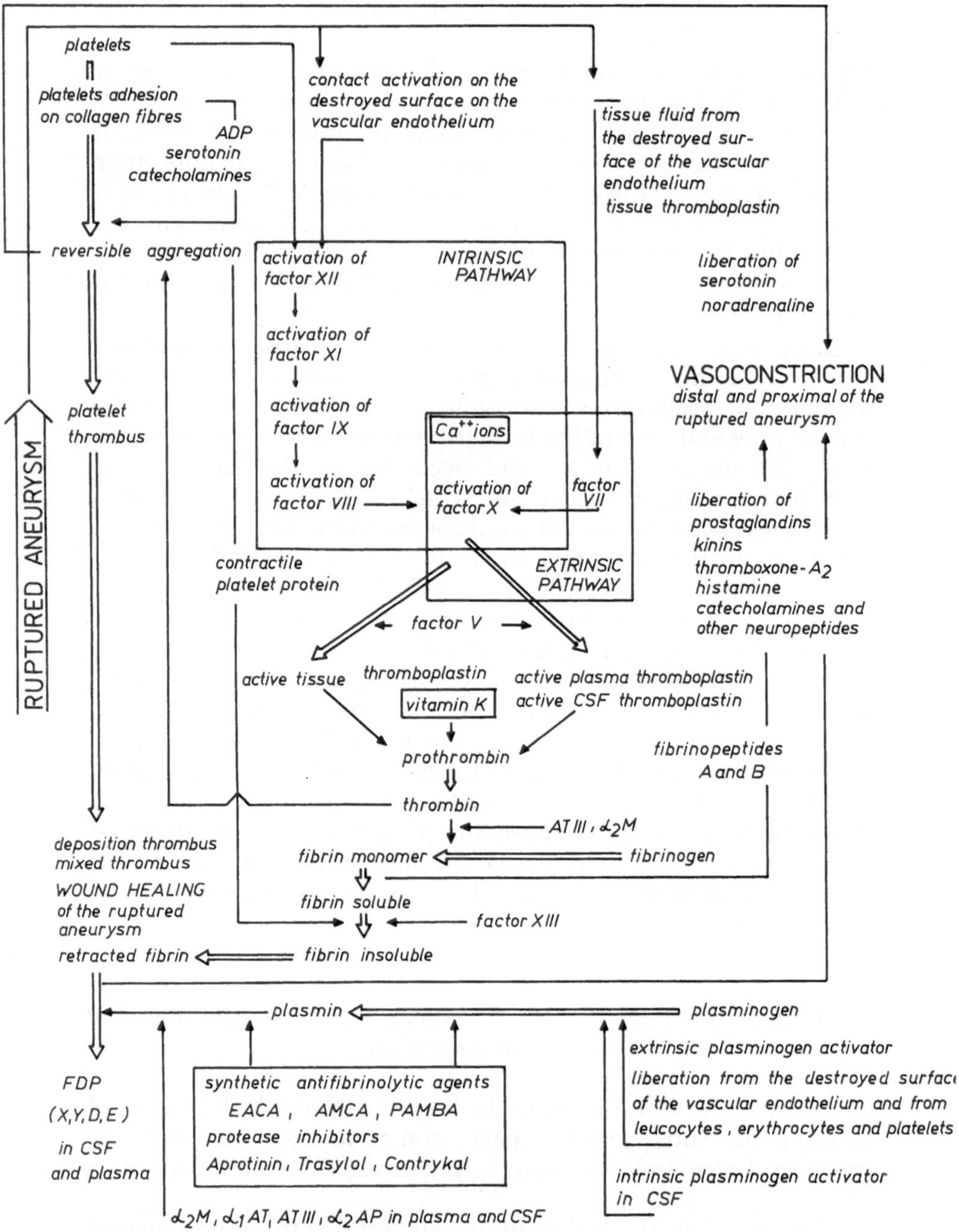

Fig. 2. Schematic representation of the coagulation and fibrinolysis pathway in connection with the formation and dissolution of the mixed thrombus. Effect on →. Formation of ⇒. Therapeutic effect ⌐

The thrombin immediately arising from the prothrombin by extrinsinc pathway activation, is on the one hand, responsible for the rapid formation of fibrin on the margin of the wound and on the other hand, for the occurrence of the activated blood thromboplastin of the intrinsic system (see Fig. 2)[18, 26, 154, 192].

In the case of free thrombin present locally the change from F I into the fibrin molecule takes place. By means of this reaction the integrity of the aneurysm is restored in the first place.

Under the influence of the aggregating platelets the mixed clotting or fibrin deposition thrombus will then be retracted. Obliteration of the aneurysm takes place by a concentrically stratified thrombus mixed and infiltrated with fibroblasts and capillaries. Now the strength of the aneurysmal fibrin deposition thrombus can withstand a slight change in the pressure and lumen, without being detached from the connective tissue.

Not until the transformation into fibrillary connective tissue with hyalinized portions of tissue is the removal of the thrombus almost completed. Formation of endothelium on the surface of the thrombus, from the neighbouring intact cells of the vessel wall concludes the reparative tissue response[32, 42, 102, 105, 159, 213, 237, 241, 302].

Causal changes in the haemostasis are comparatively rare causes of a primary or recurrent SAH. This includes patients with factor I, VIII, IX deficiency, v. Willebrand's syndrome, XI, XII and XIII deficiency, platelet cerebral haemorrhage, leucoses, SAH during anticoagulant or platelet inhibitory therapy and induced hyperfibrinolysis[24, 88, 145, 166, 167, 176, 251, 292].

Selective coagulation analyses in the plasma facilitate the prognosis of subsequent disturbances in aneurysmal wound healing. If pathological values are shown to be present, causal treatment is imperative. Interventions in form of compensating the coagulation defects or blockage of increased enzyme activities should favourably influence the outlook, course and prognosis of an SAH.

Although in case of an aetiologically unelucidated SAH, generalized disturbances of haemostasis have frequently been specified as the cause[53, 166, 292], the latter should be left out of consideration as regards the majority of recurrent SAH. For that reason the many insufficiently consolidated aneurysmal fibrin deposition thrombi in SAH patients do not correlate with the comparatively rarely occurring generalized acute and latent haemorrhagic syndromes. Even if in most of the patients the source of bleeding is temporarily occluded at the time of admission to hospital, the coagulation analyses will nevertheless remain of paramount importance for the diagnosis by exclusion. Patients with SAH, whatsoever the cause might be, should without exception show normal coagulation values.

5.4. Fibrinolytic Reactions and Dissolution of a Thrombus After Bleeding of an Aneurysm

Due to the fact that the aneurysm wall almost exclusively consists of thicker intima and adventitia, and that the plasminogen activator activity predominantly occurs in the vasa vasorum, with each aneurysmal bleeding tissue plasminogen activators are being set free. A fibrinolytic reaction released by these proteins may lead to the redissolving of the thrombus in the ruptured aneurysm.

Hassler and Fodstad[91,92] have demonstrated that the plasminogen activators occur predominantly in the minute adventitial vessels and in the endothelium in rupture cerebral saccular aneurysms. In the total balance of the plasminogen activator activity consideration should be given to the reactions caused by damage to the adjacent brain tissue and pia mater by the blood entering the subarachnoid space (stimulus caused by foreign bodies). These reactions likewise set free extrinsic plasminogen activators (tissue-type)[126,147,268,269]. Furthermore, the embedded erythrocytes, platelets and granulocytes disintegrate during the change over from a mixed to a hyaline thrombus[23,110]. With this proteolytic reaction in association with the surrounding tissue, the embedded erythrocytes, leucocytes and platelets produce, in addition to the plasminogen bound to the fibrin by adsorption, another part of tissue plasminogen activators[141,267].

Hence, for the overall assessment of the inner and the outer lysis of the thrombus the knowledge about the plasminogen activator activity in cerebral vessels is as significant[32,91,92,110,271] as the understanding of the effect by the fibrinolytically active blood-stained CSF[64,65,101,112,114,184,262,268], or the extent of the fibrinolytic reaction at the proliferation phase of wound healing[21,23,259,212,258,267,285].

The mixed thrombus in an aneurysm may thus be destroyed by an inner and outer fibrinolytic reaction (Fig. 3).

According to Ambrus and Marcus[6] and Tovi[271], part of the plasminogen is adsorbed to polymerizing fibrin, and transformed into plasmin by activators which are already in the thrombus, or enter the thrombus by diffusion[34,38,285]. Moreover, the partially formed inactive plasmin inhibitor complexes dissociate in the blood

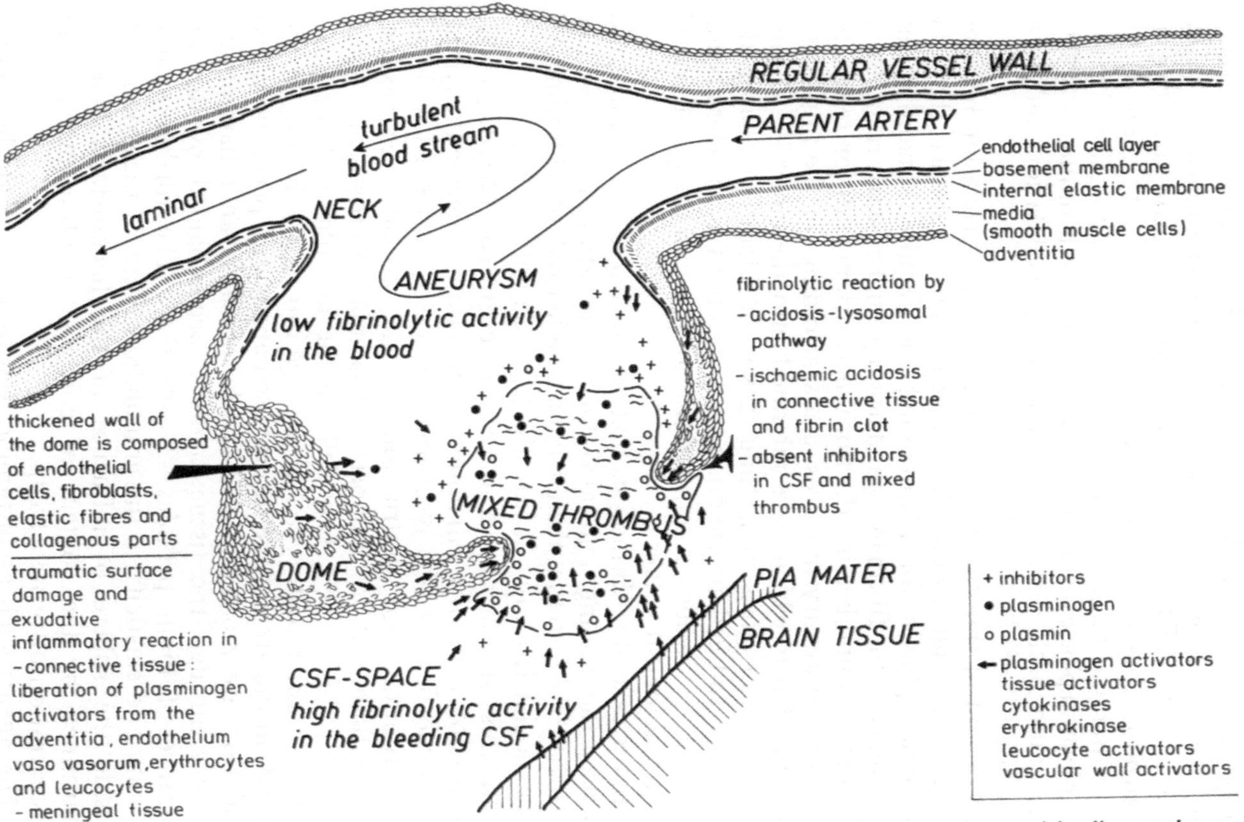

Fig. 3. Author's concept of the interplay between rCBF, coagulation, fibrinolytic factors and wound healing at the onset and during the further course of SAH

and CSF in the presence of fibrin. This is due to the fact that plasmin has a greater affinity for fibrin than for its inhibitors[6,38,39,79]. The destruction of the thrombus by an extrinsic and intrinsic lysis[105,271] is induced because antiplasmins (α_2M, α_2AP, α_1AT, AT III) do not adhere to the fibrin thrombus by adsorption, but they are squeezed out in the retraction of the depositing and mixed thrombus[173]. The effects produced by this free plasmin phase inside and outside the mixed thrombus[18,26,169,173] may cause both a disturbed phase of consolidation and total dissolution[149,267,285].

The aim of this chapter is to describe the correlation between haemostasis and wound healing in such a manner that the individual phases for maintaining the required quantity and persistence of the fibrin in wound healing can be clearly recognized. In normal wound healing the fibrin network in addition to sealing the ruptured aneurysm serves as a scaffolding for the fibroblasts and angioblasts which have migrated into the clot[14,241]. During the further progress of healing (tissue proliferation phase), the fibrin has fulfilled its function and is subject to a degradation reaction[258,267], whose onset, power and duration must not exceed the physiological values.

In the case of a fibrinolysis that has started too early and is too intense, the sealing and also the proliferation phase will be disturbed[244,267], so that there will be a higher risk of rebleeding[15,21] in particular from the fifth to the tenth day after SAH.

In this statement we have not even considered so far, the possible exudative inflammatory reaction alongside the lymph and tissue fissures, the lysosomal processes associated with tissue irritation and destruction in the wound area, exudation, inflammeation, acidosis, ischaemia, necrosis and catabolism[16,37,102,131,159,250]. Especially in the last phase of the post-traumatic inflammatory vessel damage during the healing of the wound, in the area of the thrombosed aneurysm, permeation and exudation are most marked. The latter cause an inflammatory oedema through the tissue acidosis, accompanied by the appearance of kinin peptides[16,52,77,191,192,250]. The further wound stability and elasticity in the granulation tissue of the wound are outside the sphere of influence of the haemostasis and are determined by the content of collagenous fibre and by the concentration of proteoglycan.

The agents such as histamine, serotonin and catecholamines (Fig. 2) influencing the regulation of the capillary permeation and wound healing are not considered here. However, they are not clearly distinguishable from the bradykinin effects of the kallikrein-kinin pathway on which antifibrinolytic or antiprotease treatment with aprotinin likewise has an effect[77, 169, 250].

Considering the significance of proteases in wound healing of thrombosed aneurysms, the regulation of the proteolytic pathway, to obtain a mean level, has theoretically been substantiated and is thus therapeutically necessary[16, 64, 171, 191, 268, 278].

6. Pathophysiological Changes in Coagulation and Fibrinolysis in SAH

6.1. Follow-Up Studies of Coagulation Factors in Plasma

It is known that after bleeding into the subarachnoid space far-reaching changes in coagulation may occur sporadically[88, 94, 152, 279]. Hence, a follow-up study about the relationships as they prevail in haemostasis is required in order possibly to initiate a substitution therapy or an effective systemic haemostyptic therapy[168, 204, 268, 305]. The platelets especially and the fibrinogen, which together deliver the anatomical substrate for the rapid obliteration of a ruptured aneurysm should, together with the extrinsic and intrinsic coagulation pathway, show no departure from the usual pattern.

On the basis of the research activities by Matsunaga[177], Ettinger[53], Tovi[268] and Fodstad[64] who have altogether determined nearly all coagulation factors after aneurysmal SAH, follow-up studies on SAH in a group of patients were once more performed relating to the most important factors during hospital treatment which extended over several weeks (see Fig. 4). The high frequency of recurrent SAH within the first three weeks led us again to check coagulation after primary SAH.

The increased coagulability which was found[53, 177] can only be partly confirmed. It seems to lead to wrong estimations when the individual coagulation values in SAH patients of a different category, grade I–V, by Hunt and Hess[122] in an asymmetric scatter are graphically plotted as mean values. Single curves or point clouds in the diagram would be representative on their own, but they almost completely diminish the value of the survey.

According to Fig. 4[108] the platelet count, thromboplastin time and fibrinogen value are subject to changes which after some delay settle themselves down to the normal basic position. The changes of the factors II, V, VIII, recalcification time, platelet count are inconsistently assessed by the authors[53, 108, 177]. There is agreement with that AT III decrease and a negative ethanol gelation test. Both a marked increase in fibrinogen and the PTT values point to hypercoagulability.

The cause of the wide scatter of the coagulation values is predominantly due to the variable test group, the number of patients of different degrees of severity of SAH according to Hunt

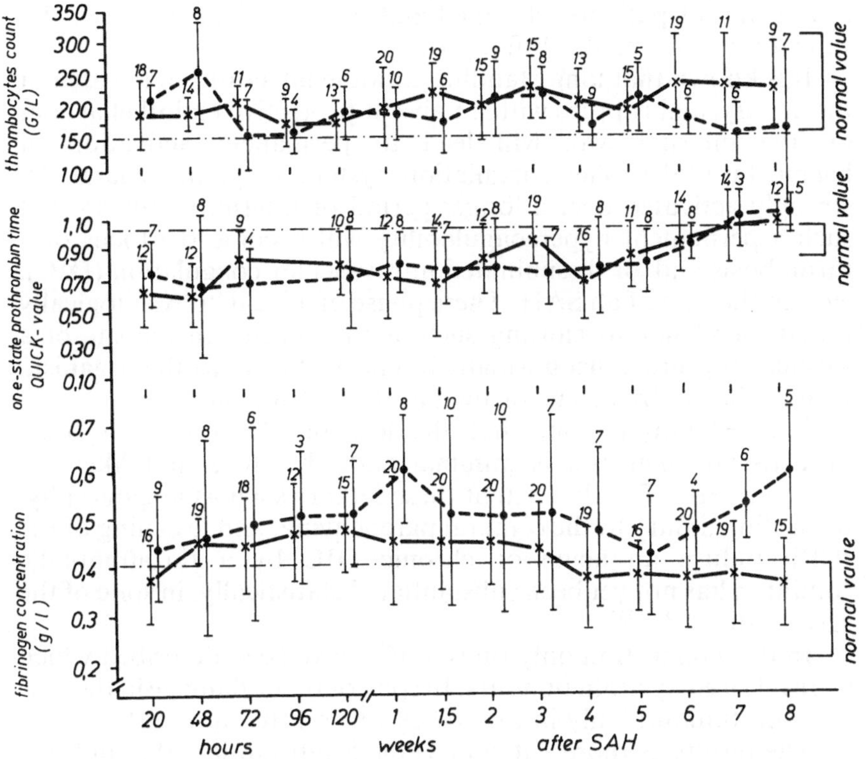

Fig. 4. Follow-up studies of coagulation factors in plasma after SAH. Mean value curve and ($\bar{x} \pm s$) of the SAH group of patients with no fatal outcome (continuous line), and fatal outcome (interrupted line)

and Hess[122], and should not be overestimated in the total assessment.

Coagulation abnormalities, induced in the course of an SAH, however, must have therapeutic consequences.

From the onset up to the third week of an SAH, increased fibrinogen values have again and again been worked out as statistically significant ($P < 0.001$), as compared to the initial value regarded as normal (< 20 hours value after onset of bleeding)[53,108,177]. The tendency of the fibrinogen to return to normal is in agreement with the healing phase[108]. Nevertheless, just before the death of SAH patients there will be a marked increase, in view of the fact that fibrinogen represents an acute-phase protein.

The response curves separately plotted in Fig. 4 with reference to a group of patients who died and to those who survived, else show only some slight differences.

It is known that long-standing endothelial lesions in the area of the aneurysmal rupture with an absent protective endothelial coat on the internal wall will lead to permanent activation of haemostasis[39,121]. The coagulation system may, in general, be strongly activated over a longer period or intermittently, so that such a permanent hypercoagulability will become the focus of a thrombosis and/or dissiminated intravascular coagulation (DIC), even in the case of an SAH. These phase of a local "physiologically raised" tendency to clotting such as may occur on the site of a vascular rupture, must normally be checked in a healthy organism without harm, by means of the antithrombin system.

Loew[164] pointed out that the loss of blood from a basal intracranial aneurysm is minimal and, therefore, not likely to initiate a DIC. To what extent these factors such as angiography, rebleeding, injury to the cerebral parenchyma, and lessening of the rCBF induce an acute or chronic DIC by a thrombophilic condition has not yet been substantiated statistically, in spite of the case studies[36,213,232].

In this connection only those DICs have been described which were released by brain tumours. In spite of tissue damage in the case of brain tumours only in rare cases was a DIC induced[176,192].

The results as represented in Table 5 substantiate that in SAH patients no intravascular coagulopathy has occurred as an initial phase of DIC at the time of bleeding or in its further course.

The typical manifestations of DIC, not evident in our cases investigated during and after SAH (platelet count < 100 G/l, F I < 0.1 g/l, AT III < 0.25 g/l, FDP > 0.01 g/l and positive ethanol gelation test), therefore, exclude DIC[18,44,305].

In this connection the relationship between thrombosed aneurysms and cerebral thrombosis manifested in situ, thromboembolic diseases and cerebral infarction, must be pointed out[62,78,121,174,192]. Recent studies by Mettinger and Egberg[183] substantiate an altered haemostasis in ischaemic cerebrovascular disease with abnormalities in factor VIII, AT III, α-2 AP, platelet ADP and vascular plasminogen activators (tissue type).

Table 5. *Representative Diagnostic Values for the Exclusion of DIC*

Methods	Normal values	Analytical values in SAH patients (n = 30)
One-stage prothrombin time (Quick value)	1.0–0.80	0.90 ± 0.30
Platelet count	155–300 G/l	see response curves Fig. 4
Fibrinogen concentration	2.2–4.1 g/l	see response curves Fig. 4
Ethanol gelation test	negative	negative
Factors II, V, VIII, and X activities	normal	sporadically reduced
AT III concentration	0.25–0.35 g/l	0.26 ± 0.05
FDP-D concentration	< 5 mg/l	< 5 mg/l (n = 25) > 15 mg/l (n = 5)

6.2. Follow-Up Studies of Fibrinolytic Factors in Plasma

From the onset of a SAH, the fibrinolytic activity from blood and fluorescein-isothiocyanate-labelled fibrin indicator substrate are recorded over the plasma lysis time and euglobulin lysis time.

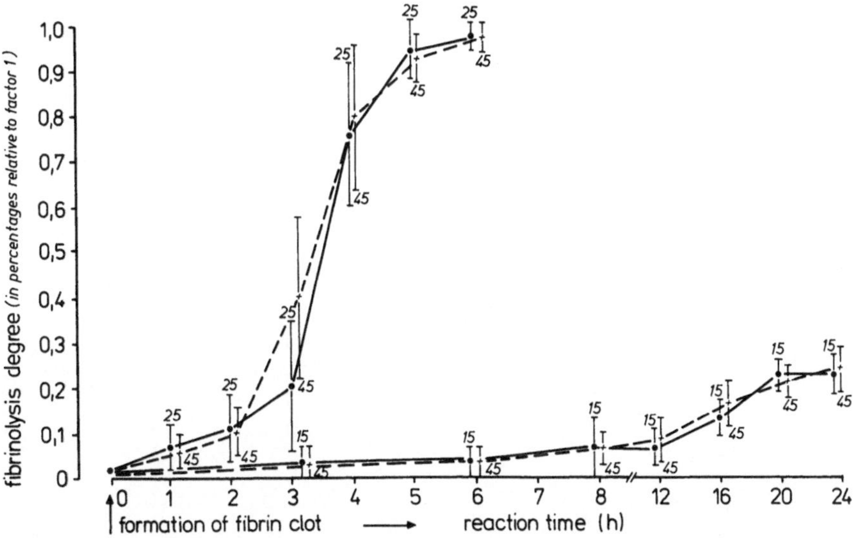

Fig. 5. Plasma and euglobulin lysis time. Follow-up studies for the assessment of fibrinolytic activities. Blood was withdrawn from SAH patients 24, 72 and 120 hours after the bleeding

The mean value curves of all analytical values in volunteers (———) (n = 25) and SAH patients (----) (n = 15) showed no significant differences ($p > 0.05$) (Fig. 5), neither with reference to the steep euglobulin lysis curve nor as regards the flat course of the plasma lysis time curve. Fibrinolytic activity at the phase of bleeding and in the subsequent course could not be detected. The concentration of plasminogen remained within normal limits. On average, the increased fibrinogen values were 0.45 g/l. Noteworthy are the serum FDP values of > 10 mg/l identified in five out of 30 cases. They were detected solely in patients who had died within ten days of their SAH[105]. Whether there is any prognostic importance to be attached to these findings, in the absence of symptoms of DIC, is kept in reserve in favour of other examinations[64, 65, 105, 268, 272]. No indications of thromboembolic disease were seen at post-mortem.

7. Treatment of SAH

7.1. The Status of Conservative Treatment

Before it becomes possible to introduce a pattern of treatment on the basis of the results of investigations, some fundamental considerations about conservative treatment are necessary.

1. Conservative treatment is not a substitute for the surgical removal of the source the bleeding of which as the sole causal measure should be taken as early as possible.

2. Conservative treatment fills in the time before the operation and becomes the sole alternative when the bleeding source cannot be located angiographically or with CT scan, or when an operation is contra-indicated.

3. The targets of conservative treatment, as recognized today, apart from normalizing and stabilizing the disturbed cerebral metabolism, the blood pressure and the rCBF, are in particular to promote aneurysmal clot formation, to inhibit delayed reactions and thus to prevent rebleeding.

7.2. Treatment to Promote Clotting

In case of SAH the relevance of immediately testing the coagulation functions, for the exclusion of causal disturbances of haemostasis in the plasma, is beyond doubt.

For the control of disturbances, occurring at the aneurysmal phase of wound healing, several Quick values, PTT, platelet count, fibrinogen and FDP will suffice[108].

Reductions in the Quick values < 0.8 after SAH can be adjusted daily to the normal value of 1.0 by means of 10 to 20 mg of vitamin K_1. Such a procedure is justified from a therapeutic point of view, because any kind of wound healing—even in cases of a cerebral vascular lesion—presupposes optimum values in the coagulation pathway in order to prevent rebleeding, possibly the result of an existing tendency to bleed[110].

Apart from the administration of ascorbic acid which prevents failure in mucopolysaccharide formation in connective tissue elements of the blood vessel wall, it can be dispensed with other agents such as highly polymerized pectins despite earlier suggestions to the fact that they have no haemostatic effect[105, 110]. The high values of intrinsic thromboplastin in CSF as compared to plasma, as well as the liberating quantities of extrinsic thromboplastin in cases of a traumatic cerebral vessel wall and brain damage only sporadically produce a low hypercoagulability[17, 105].

This result by no means entitles one to expect a favourable effect on the wound healing. The rare cases of thrombophilia associated with a SAH from which no anticoagulatory consequences result, are faced by the much higher risk of a local fibrinolytic tendency to haemorrhages in the area of wound healing between blood, vessel wall and CSF.

7.3. Antifibrinolytic Therapy

In case of a vascular lesion the extrinsic coagulation pathway must, at least locally, dominate the instrinsic coagulation pathway in order to maintain the integrity of the site of rupture in the vessel, and to ensure rapid and secure formation and subsequent consolidation of the haemostatic plug. From clinical experience, however, it can be shown that a high percentage of SAH patients is affected with the prognostically unfavourable recurrent SAH which, to some extent, can be attributed to a local disturbance of haemostasis in the thrombosed aneurysm[64, 110, 268].

From the reference material[2, 5, 7, 21, 31, 33, 35, 40, 54, 59, 60, 64—73, 80, 82—84, 86, 95, 105, 129, 133, 135, 136, 138, 158, 160, 166, 171, 179, 190, 195—199, 203, 213, 218, 221, 225, 228, 239, 245, 247—249, 252, 268, 270, 271, 273, 275, 277, 280, 282, 283, 285, 286, 289, 290, 297] it can be gathered that SAH patients have been treated both with synthetic antifibrinolytic agents and sporadically with naturally occurring protease inhibitors, or by combinations of these two drugs with the aim of strengthening the mixed thrombus at the site of rupture[10, 11, 23, 42, 50, 92, 149, 210, 212, 267], and thus reducing the high risk of rebleeding during the first weeks after haemorrhage[64, 105, 268]. Such treatment is frequently used in cases of SAH before and after surgical intervention on the aneurysm with the aim of performing the intervention without excessive loss of blood, by blocking the high concentration of plasminogen activator (tissue-type) in the dura mater[202].

According to Markwardt[169], the effect of all synthetic antifibrinolytica (EACA, AMCA, PAMBA) consists not only in an

Table 6. *Pharmacokinetic Data on Antifibrinolytics in Man.* KTU = Kallikrein-inactivator units; ATrU = antitrypsin unit

Drugs	Active agent concentration (mg/l) in whole blood	Half-life (minutes) t ½ in plasma	Maintenance dose in cases of SAH
ε-Aminocaproic acid (EACA) Epsicapron (Kabi) EAC (Berlin-chemistry) Amicar (Lederle) Capramol (Laboratoire Choay)	100–130	88–127	5 g every 4–6 hours by mouth
Trans-4-aminomethyl-cyclohexane-carboxylic acid-(1) (t-AMCHA) tranexamic acid Ugurol (Bayer) Cyclocapron (Kabi) Transamin (Daiichi Seiyaku Co. Ltd.)	> 10	80	3 g every 12 hours by mouth 3 g every 12 hours intravenous injection
p-Aminomethylbenzoic acid PAMBA (AWD) Gumbix (Kali)	> 15	52–71	0.25 g every 4–6 hours oral and 0.05 g intrathecal every 36 hours
Protease inhibitors (Aprotinin) Trasylol (Bayer) Iniprol (Laboratoire Choay) Contrykal (AWD)	20	119–240	500,000 KIU every 8 hours, 60,000 ATrU every 6 hours intravenous injection

immediate antifibrinolytic activity, but also in a competitive inhibition of the plasminogen-activating proteins (Table 6).

EACA in high therapeutic doses has a similar effect to AMCA and PAMBA and is practically non-toxic [43]. The partially disturbed BBB function represents a barrier only to a limited extent when a quantity of EACA up to 36 g is given [158, 216]. Starting from the demand that synthetic antifibrinolytic agents should reach the necessary active concentrations, even in the CSF space, if the treatment is to be adequate, such quantities of EACA must be given which would hardly be tolerated by the SAH patients, and which also present marked stress to the kidney function[171].

For that reason the synthetic antifibrinolytic agents such as AMCA and PAMBA which are on average ten times more effective, are to be preferred to EACA[43,169,173].

The AMCA levels in CSF in the case of SAH patients, detected solely by Tovi *et al.*[268,273,275] after repeated continuous oral administration of 6 g AMCA daily, do not confirm that tranexamic acid generally overcomes the BBB. The reduced frequently even abolished barrier function within the marginal area between the capillary endothelium and glial tissue in this instance or in other cases permits a limited passage of the AMCA drug into the CSF spaces. Tovi[268] and Fodstad[63,64] have estimated the concentration in the CSF as being from 4.8 to 6.0 mg/l, so that despite high oral doses of AMCA the concentration remained far below the required optimum active amount of > 10 mg/l.

In the same way PAMBA as a non-lipophile drug, does not penetrate into the CSF spaces at all, or only to a slight degree—a finding that is dealt with in chapter 8.1.

Another variant of AFT is the use of the combination of protease inhibitors and comparatively low doses of 2 to 3 g of AMCA, for single drug therapy[20,21,239,249,254,278].

Naturally occurring inhibitors of the proteolytic enzyme Aprotinin (Trasylol, Iniprol, Contrykal)[169] also inhibit the formation of plasmin, and bind the active plasmin which is already present. They do not penetrate the normal BBB[130] but only a highly disturbed one[278,303] and in addition to their antifibrinolytic and antiproteolytic effect on wound healing[175] they also exert a positive influence on the oedema caused by the SAH, by inhibition of the Kallikrein[21,249,278]. On the strength of the reaction course (cerebral vasospasm, reduced rCBF, hypoxia) cells damaged by acidosis, liberate kininpeptides, the effect of which should be inhibited with Aprotinin as far as possible[52,249,293]. Aprotinin also inhibits liberation of vasoactive agents[250], and by blocking the kinin pathway it shows an antishock effect[21,52,191,250,278]. In addition to the poor coagulation-inhibiting effect[173] the possible anaphylactic reaction[219] might be the reason why protease inhibitors, in comparison, have scarcely been used at all.

In most of the publications it has remained an open question whether the EACA and AMCA levels in the blood reached by oral or parenteral administration will suffice to attain the required concentration of antifibrinolytic active agent in the CSF and the aneurysmal connective tissue by the steady state and the concentration gradient which emerges when the BBB function is disturbed.

The majority of the statistically interpreted results obtained with EACA, AMCA and PAMBA, however, make this evident as controlled studies[2, 5, 33, 35, 59, 65, 67, 70, 82, 179, 180, 196, 217, 225, 239, 245, 290], or as uncontrolled studies[2, 40, 41, 68, 94, 189, 190, 195, 197, 198, 203, 221, 247, 270, 271, 273, 280], in terms of the therapeutic result. Moreover, significant variations as to the untreated patients had been recorded as the result of treatment, not only as regards the frequency of the occurrence of recurrent SAH, but also with regard to the survival rate.

In a comparison made with the statistically interpreted AFT results the view is confirmed that pathophysiological and anatomical risk factors which cannot be influenced, such as

(i) hypertension or short-term variations in hypertension,
(ii) size, shape and location of the ruptured aneurysm,
(iii) intra-aneurysmal turbulence,
(iv) cerebral vascular spasm accompanied by ischaemia,
(v) a transition into meningo-cerebral haemorrhage of a progressive character [classification of patients with intracranial aneurysms, category grade IV and V by Hunt and Hess[122]] may disguise the antifibrinolytic and thus the fibrin stabilizing effect in the overall result.

Likewise an inadequate antifibrinolytic level around the thrombosed aneurysm and the retrospective evaluation of a too small number of SAH patients, particularly in earlier publications, is often the cause of erroneous assessments.

Since it is only a question of a multi-factor process involving many different influencing factors, only comprehensive controlled, randomized controlled trials or double blind studies are relevant for statistical interpretation. There are certain factors which can be influenced in such studies and these are crucial in assessing a positive or negative beneficial antifibrinolytic effect on rebleeding and mortality, which is statistically significant[65, 220]. These factors include such things as the individual assignment to the classifications by Hunt and Hess[122] and Botterell[29, 213], which are only comparable with each other to a certain extent, statistical interpretation and comparison of groups too small in number, or groups of differently itemized maxima of the number of patients in the grades I to V, AFT with different EACA, AMCA, PAMBA and Aprotinin drug levels, combination therapy—AFT plus hypotension, conservative pre-operative and postoperative comparative studies performed by various clinics, and different error probability.

Thus it is not difficult to grasp that some contributions reporting no therapeutic result[7, 80, 83, 84, 86, 135—137, 218, 228, 248], and some replies[73, 133, 160, 282, 297] are known as well.

The results which show no effect on rebleeding do not necessarily justify another lumbar puncture, as the deterioration in the clinical picture may be due purely to cerebral ischaemia.

8. Antifibrinolytic Treatment of SAH with PAMBA

8.1. Oral Administration

The investigations carried out within the setting of a planned oral or i.v. treatment with PAMBA are directed at finding out whether the drug brings under control

(i) the normal BBB function,

(ii) the pathologically changed BBB function due to inflammatory reactions in CNS,

(iii) the severely disturbed BBB function in cases of intracranial bleeding,

and also reaches the therapeutically required level in the CSF.

By giving due consideration to all pharmacokinetic and biological factors it is necessary to attain EACA levels of > 100 μg/ml, AMCA levels of > 10 μg/ml and PAMBA levels of from 15 to 25 μg/ml continuously at the site of action[9, 116], in order to meet the requirement for an 80% inhibition of fibrinolytic activity[9, 169, 173].

The patients listed in Table 7 had been given 6 g of PAMBA orally in accordance with the factors known for PAMBA such as invasion, half-life and possible permeation, 120 minutes before the

Table 7. *Determination of Permeation of the Drug PAMBA into the CSF Spaces.* Two hours before lumbar puncture the patients were given 6 g of PAMBA by mouth

Groups	Number (n)	PAMBA concentration in CSF	
Patients with normal BBB function	64	63 patients 1 patient	< 1 μg/ml 3 μm/ml
Patients with disturbed BBB function	30	28 patients 2 patients	< 1 μg/ml 3–10 μg/ml
SAH patients with severely disturbed BBB function	20	12 patients 8 patients	< 1 μg/ml 3–15 μg/ml

withdrawal of CSF, in order to determine the maximum PAMBA level reached in the CSF.

The results obtained show[116] that a necessary PAMBA level of > 15 µg/ml in CSF even with high concentrations of > 0.5 g of PAMBA/l in the plasma and with severely disturbed BBB function in case of SAH is achieved either not at all, or only to some extent.

The alternative in our opinion should not be a still higher dosage which would induce side effects[45, 56, 69, 103, 120, 171, 231, 280, 299] but should rather be intrathecal instillation.

8.2. Intrathecal Administration

Due to varied enzymatic and pharmacokinetic reactions, intrathecal therapy requires, as compared to the central compartment blood, a limited range of concentration of the drug[142]. Antifibrinolytic treatment with PAMBA for inhibiting the endogenous and exogenous fibrinolysis in the clot which occludes the aneurysm is no exception, here. Due to the fact that the dissolution of the fibrin clot takes place in the wound area between the blood, vessel wall and CSF, the antifibrinolytic effect in the plasma cannot be sufficient on its own to prevent fibrinolysis of the fibrin thrombus deposited from the CSF boundary side. For that reason a sufficient concentration of active agents in the CSF also, is a requirement for adequate treatment.

In our opinion two factors determine the use of intrathecal administration.

Firstly: An improvement in the concept of therapy by maintaining a continuous concentration of active agents in the CSF without stressing the central compartment of blood, and secondly: if the antifibrinolytic agents given by the oral or parenteral route enter in quantities which because of the BBB function must be regarded as too low, or as ineffective metabolites in the CSF space.

Thus, in spite of high dosages of 48 g of EACA/day and 9 g of AMCA/day, for instance only 6 mg of AMCA/l were found in the CSF[64, 86]. This value is far below the required active limit of > 10 mg/l, and produces nothing but an essentially lower inhibitor effect.

With lumbar puncture, at least such a quantity of CSF must be withdrawn as is necessary to re-inject as the volume required for the PAMBA level[105, 142]. By this exchange, no or just an insignificant variation in CSF pressure will be produced and also the circulation of the drug in the CSF space will be encouraged[54, 85, 142, 226].

The circulation in general present under SAH conditions[140], after repeated lumbar instillation, permits a PAMBA level, even in the subarachnoid space, of > 10 mg/l[106]. This evidence has been confirmed in a test series 12 hours after a lumbar injection, by the withdrawal of CSF during the intraventricular measuring of CSF pressure, suboccipital puncture, or in the course of the operative treatment of the aneurysm[106]. The pre-albumin proteins to a large extent still existing in blood-stained CSF are also reliable data for the circulation of CSF[47].

The most favourable results obtained (Table 8) in earlier animal experiments (15 dogs of 25 kg each)[109] on the ascertained penetration, distribution, half-life and compatibility of PAMBA in CSF should be transferred for clinical therapeutic application only with some reservations. Apart from the ascertained $t_{1/2}$ values, with some certainty but also by these animal experiments, any damaging effects on the brain from intrathecal administration would have been detectable. With amounts of PAMBA which are 250 times higher than the necessary therapeutic dosage, generalized tonic-clonic spasms or localized myoclonia have developed, which could be controlled with diazepam[109].

The difference between the $t_{1/2}$ values in plasma (60 minutes) and CSF (540 minutes) must be attributed to the selective effect of the BBB function as against the non-lipophile PAMBA drug, as well as the absent biotransformation in CSF.

The PAMBA concentrations incubated in CSF for the determination of the biotransformation by way of a
(i) plasmalysis test activated by streptokinase (n = 25) and
(ii) euglobulin lysis test (n = 20)
were compared in their inhibitory effect with the same amounts of PAMBA dissolved in buffer[105]. This reaction mixture permits an assessment of possible inactivation of the PAMBA by an enzymatic N-acetylation reaction taking place in the CSF.

The results showed no significant differences ($p > 0.05$), so that the hypothesis of an absent extrahepatic biotransformation in CSF is confirmed[105].

The decrease in concentration after intrathecal administration of PAMBA and, therefore, the duration of action is predominantly dependent on the CSF $t_{1/2}$ value which includes the diffusion rate through the CSF blood barrier and also the distribution in the extracellular and intracellular space of the brain.

Due to the fact that the results obtained with intrathecal instillation in an animal can be transferred to man only with some

Table 8. *Factors in Intrathecal PAMBA Therapy*

Factors involved	Animals (dogs) n = 15	SAH patients n = 25, single measurements n = 65
Amount of CSF	$\bar{x}$ = 10 ml (8–12 ml)	$\bar{x}$ = 200 ml (170–230 ml)
Amount of PAMBA instilled i.th. (absolute)	10 mg 33 mg	20 mg 40 mg 50 mg
In case of an assumed normal distribution in CSF	1,000 µg/ml 3,300 µg/ml	100 µg/ml 200 µg/ml 250 µg/ml
Overdosage relative to the therapeutically effective level	75-fold for half life determination 250-fold for the determination of side-effects	7.7-fold 15.4-fold 19.2-fold
Antifibrinolytically effective level	≧ 15 µg/ml	≧ 15 µg/ml
Half-life in CSF	160 minutes	540 minutes
Duration until the drug concentration is below normal	17 hours related to 1,000 mg	36 hours related to 50 g

reservations, because unforeseen total effects or side effects may occur according to the chemical structure and the mechanism of action, at the beginning intrathecal administration was fixed at a comparatively low level, at 20 mg to be slowly increased and finally fixed at 50 mg (Table 8).

First the drug was injected only into patients who showed clinically the most severe forms of recurrent SAH. However, all of them showed an unfavourable outcome.

The CSF withdrawn under clinical indications allows a graphic representation of the half-life for PAMBA of 540 minutes, valid only when there is disturbed BBB function (Fig. 6). Another 40 concentration-time curves have confirmed that after 36 hours the PAMBA level was below the detection limit of < 5 µg/ml, from which somewhat smaller half-lives than 540 minutes can be deduced.

From the elimination rate thus determined, it follows that for treatment 50 mg of PAMBA should be given intrathecally every 30 to 40 hours, in order to meet the need not to be below the therapeutically required concentration over a longer period, and not to be within the possible toxic ranges of concentration. No toxic effects due to cumulative action was observed. Clinical observation

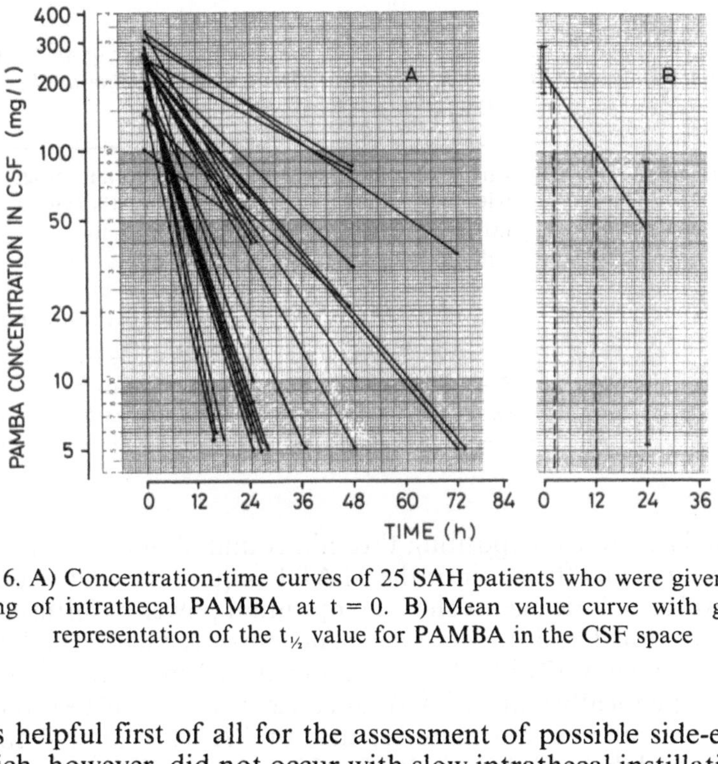

Fig. 6. A) Concentration-time curves of 25 SAH patients who were given 20 to 50 mg of intrathecal PAMBA at t = 0. B) Mean value curve with graphic representation of the $t_{1/2}$ value for PAMBA in the CSF space

was helpful first of all for the assessment of possible side-effects which, however, did not occur with slow intrathecal instillation of the drug and with pressure compensation when giving the injection.

The good results obtained with AFT in CSF were confirmed diagnostically in further withdrawals of CSF, by lowering the FDP level with reference to the therapeutically unaffected blood-stained CSF[64, 105, 180, 268]. Seventy-five per cent of the total CSF in SAH patients treated intrathecally showed amounts of FDP of just < 5 µg/ml during the second withdrawal (Table 9). Generally confirmed and represented in the studies by Fodstad[64, 65, 71] and Maurice-Williams[180] is the correlation between the high FDP values in CSF and the progressive course of an SAH.

The morphologic findings with ruptured aneurysms substantiate the inhibited fibrinolytic activity despite the post-mortem fibrinolysis, so that the vascular lesion of occluding fibrin deposits can be easily recognized at the autopsy. There were none of the usual pathological-anatomical appearances, showing bleeding extending over the surface on the base of the brain, but there were thrombotic deposits near to the site of rupture[97].

Table 9. *The Decrease in the FDP Concentration as an Indicator of an Inhibited Fibrinolytic Reaction in CSF in SAH Patients Classified According to Hunt and Hess (Grade II and III)*

SAH patients	First CSF withdrawal with subsequent i.th. PAMBA instillation of 50 mg	Second and other CSF withdrawals after 24 to 96 hours with subsequent i.th. PAMBA instillation of 50 mg
FDP determination $n = 50$	$\bar{x} = 20.2$ µg/ml $(\bar{x} \pm s)$ 10.0–30.4	$\bar{x} = 2.2$ µg/ml $(\bar{x} \pm s)$ 0–5.2

The large fibrin depositing thrombi round about the ruptured aneurysm in an efficient intrathecal AFT require the evidence that the antifibrinolytic agents show an optimum power of diffusion in the fibrin clot. The diffusion coefficients measured with ^3H labelled compounds show (Table 10)[105, 118], that with a 3 cm large fibrin clot the therapeutically required AMCA concentrations will be attained as soon as after seven minutes, that of PAMBA after 7 to 46 minutes and that of EACA only after 720 minutes. This proves that there are considerable differences due to the different drug concentrations, although the diffusion coefficients are almost the same. Accordingly, it can be assumed on the strength of the in vitro determinations, that with in vivo intrathecal AFT the therapeutically required amount especially with AMCA and PAMBA is rapidly attained even in a large fibrin depositing thrombus. A possible endogenic fibrinolysis in the clot and connective tissue is thus prevented during the time of fibrin degradation as well as a premature and too intense fibrinolysis reaction in the phase of proliferation[6, 34, 39, 141, 169, 210, 271].

Table 10. *Determinations of Antifibrinolytic Agents After Twelve Hours to Indicate Their Powers of Diffusion.* A comparison is made between the amount of the drug in the fibrin clot and that in the incubation solution. The latter corresponds to the concentration that is produced in the CSF by the intrathecal administration of 50 mg, viz. 250 mg/l. The power of diffusion is expressed as a rate to the proportion 1. Radiochemical determination of the diffusion coefficient by using ^3H labelled EACA, AMCA and PAMBA with the capillary diffusion method. Contrykal is estimated by a synthetic chromogenic substrate

Drugs	Drug level (mg/l)	Diffusion coefficient ($cm^2 \cdot s^{-1}$)	(n)	Diffused amount as proportion to the level of the incubation solution ($\bar{x} \pm s$)	(n)	Time until the drug level is reached in the fibrin clot (minutes)
AMCA	10	($7.6 \cdot 10^{-6}$)	10	(0.90 ± 0.08)	40	7
EACA	100–130	($6.7 \cdot 10^{-6}$)	8	(0.96 ± 0.10)	40	720
PAMBA	10–25	($7.3 \cdot 10^{-6}$)	11	(0.93 ± 0.09)	40	7–40
Contrykal	20	—		(0.89 ± 0.05)	125	ca. 7

8.3. Aspects of Intrathecal Administration and Their Clinical Relevance

In the case of a SAH surgical removal of the malformation should be aimed at whenever an aneurysm or an arteriovenous angioma is demonstrated by angiography and/or in the CT scan[28, 74, 143, 213, 234, 259, 261, 288].

According to international statistics[1, 63, 94, 95, 163, 213, 258] widely differing values varying from 22 to 64%, are given for the mortality rate in cases of SAH prior to the introduction of AFT, when any surgical treatment is not possible[64, 129, 144, 188, 217]. Conservative treatment becomes the only possible alternative to avoid recurrent SAH, if the vascular malformation cannot be angiographically demonstrated, or contraindications prohibit any surgical treatment. In recent years, in addition to general measures for the control of CBF, the disturbed brain metabolism and the associated increase in the intracranial pressure, the aim of treatment was to optimise coagulation and to administer synthetic antifibrinolytic agents orally and parenterally in order to improve the healing of the ruptured aneurysm. Possible side-effects of AFT in view of an increased incidence of such as meningeal fibroses[68, 213, 300], communicating hydrocephali[68, 94, 95, 208, 213, 258, 300], cerebro-vascular ischaemic complications and peripheral thromboses[45, 56, 69, 120, 125, 127, 129, 157, 183, 211, 231, 299, 301] were considered the smaller risk up to the present as compared with the probability of rebleeding. Nevertheless, with oral/parenteral EACA or AMCA therapy in high doses there is still a higher risk of predominantly thrombotic, arteriopathic complications and meningeal fibrosis[253]. To what extent however these isolated findings[45, 56, 69, 120, 231, 299] can be solely attributed to the inhibited fibrinolytic effect in the haemostatic pathway by AFT[103, 284] has not been confirmed. Hedlund[93], for instance, using the ^{125}I fibrinogen uptake test, found no difference in the incidence of thrombosis between the patients treated with AMCA and those with placebo.

Despite the AFT, unfavourable susceptibility (sedation with neuroleptic drugs, impairment of the blood flow by a strict confinement to bed, polycythaemia, arteriosclerotic and varicose changes in the vessel wall) with an influence on the haemostasis, might promote and also induce a thrombophilic state in SAH patients. As long as it is not made clear, whether in such a pathologic constellation an AFT is contra-indicated, high oral or parenteral doses should be administered only with reservation over several weeks, at least with high-risk patients. This should be observed continously as described in cases of AFT not only because of the blocked fibrinolysis but also because of the procoagulatory side-effects by EACA and AMCA still discussed in this context[103, 173]. Likewise a reduced fibrinolytic activity resulting from low plasminogen and plasminogen activator antigen values in plasma may disturb the balance of haemostasis and manifest itself in an increased tendency to thrombosis due to depleted stores of endothelial plasminogen activator, or due to increased inhibitor levels[284].

In order to reduce the increased incidence of delayed cerebral ischaemia in AMCA-treated SAH patients, acetyl salicylic acid was given as a further measure for lowering the mortality. The double blind trial of aspirin showed no differences[181].

The prevention of subarachnoid fibrosis after SAH with intrathecal urokinase was successfully tested in animal experiments, but in our opinion it seems to be inadequate on account of the sophisticated control of the fibrinolytic process[128].

For the sake of completeness mention must be made that in the case of high EACA values in the blood there is even a dose-dependent inhibition of collagen-induced platelet aggregation, acting against coagulation. High doses of EACA (24 to 48 g/day) prolong the bleeding time and increase rebleeding and intraoperative haemorrhage in patients with SAH[83]. Most likely the side-effects by the EACA drug are different with such high doses, and can hardly be foreseen in any particular case.

When extending AFT to the combined intrathecal and oral PAMBA administration[96,97,105,170,214] in our opinion the following advantages are offered:

1. Only one hundredth of the generally necessary amount for oral medication will suffice in the case of AFT to obtain permanently the necessary therapeutic concentration in the CSF space.

2. The high oral or parenteral drug load in the case of AFT that is badly tolerated by a great many patients is no longer required, all the more so as it remains doubtful to what extent the necessary drug level in CSF is attained by these high doses.

3. The high risk of peripheral and cerebral thromboses due to a high concentration of antifibrinolytic agents in the blood no longer exists.

4. Due to the fact that there is no biotransformation of PAMBA in the CSF space, the half-life of the drug is prolonged in comparison to that in the blood. The protein values decreased by the factor 100 in CSF, increase in comparison with plasma, the freely occurring proportion of PAMBA in CSF. Pharmacokinetically from this results a higher degree of drug efficacy[47].

Intrathecal administration of 50 mg of PAMBA every 36 hours, in dependence on the BBB function of above 30 hours, provides for the required quantity of the active agent of > 10 mg/l and promotes consolidation of the aneurysmal fibrin clot as well as the wound healing proceeding from the surrounding connective tissue. In order to attain distribution of the drug in the entire subarachnoid space, at least such an amount of CSF should be withdrawn prior to PAMBA installation as is the volume to be re-injected. Several intrathecal injections within the pre-operative period together with a possible conservative therapy are required up to a maximum of 12 days for improving the healing of the wound. Rebleeding after this period is chiefly due to other factors and by no means the result of a fibrinolytic reaction, especially as an AFT beyond this time will increase the risk of a meningeal fibrosis.

Simultaneously with the intrathecal AFT the administration of only 750 mg orally, or 150 mg i.v. should suffice to inhibit any possible fibrinolytic activity in the blood which however is rather rare. A fibrinolysis of the mixed thrombus from the side by the blood stream, is thus prevented (Fig. 3).

In addition, in the case of rebleeding in CSF and from the original bleeding source the antifibrinolytic agent is available immediately[214].

The course of the disease in 25 SAH-treated intrathecally was compared with an SAH patient group without AFT but with an approximately analogous classification group according to Hunt and Hess. The two groups of patients showed no significant difference ($p > 0.05$) in their incidence rate as regards rebleeding and mortality. In contrast to this there was some difference in the following findings. Within the first 10 days after the onset of bleeding rebleedings occurred in 80% in the group without AFT, and only 28% in that of the treated patients. Mortality amounted to 12% in the group without AFT within the first 14 days, whereas all the patients having an intrathecal AFT survived. The average time of survival was 58 days in the AFT SAH group of patients, whereas the SAH patients of the control group died after 22 days on the average. The lowest rate of rebleeding and mortality was shown by the SAH patients in those cases where the intrathecal AFT was started early.

In comparison to the control group no increase in the incidence of vasospasm and fatal cerebral ischaemia, hydrocephalus obstructivus extraventricularis due to a subarachnoid fibrosis and cerebral circulatory disturbances could be confirmed. Likewise there were no supplementary reactive CSF cell variations, epileptic reactions and other side-effects in case of the intrathecal AFT. 25 other SAH patients without rebleeding and motality within the first 6 weeks after the onset of bleeding strengthen the assumption of a successful i.th. AFT. The CT scan representation did not indicate any increased incidence under i.th. AFT with reference to hydrocephalus obstructivus extraventricularis. Leska and Krupka[156] arrived at similar conclusions. They had no fatalities during the first 21 days with a group of patients treated intrathecally ($n = 31$), but a mortality rate of 47% with an untreated control group.

If the above-mentioned possible complications could be detected repeatedly in a larger group of patients under an intrathecal AFT, most likely it would be better with mild cases of SAH (classification from Hunt and Hess grade I), and without any evidence of malformation, to do without intrathecal treatment.

Generally speaking, we think it more advisable to incorporate the intrathecal AFT with PAMBA into the programme of treatment as an alternative method in addition to the combined oral and parenteral AFT with EACA and AMCA, especially because in spite of the invasive form of administration, the excellent tolerance and thus the attainment of the therapeutically required PAMBA level in the CSF justify such a procedure.

Nevertheless, a microsurgical operation that should be performed as early as possible[27, 134, 144, 161, 188, 213, 259, 261, 291, 300] should be the unique causal treatment of aneurysms. Even in those cases in which the AFT of the ruptured aneurysm with subsequent reaction of the connective tissue has led to a thrombus, this will remain a *locus minoris resistentiae*.

Summary

Among the reasons for intensified research into the CSF haemostatic pathway were the clinical case reports stating that special importance must be attached to the CSF for the high incidence of rebleeding and the intraoperative haemorrhage rate in SAH patients, which, among other things, may be regarded as the reasons for mortality. Extensive analyses of the coagulation and fibrinolysis enzyme systems were carried out and constitute the basic concept for the conservative AFT aiming at restoring to normal haemostasis and wound healing which had been disturbed by local fibrinolytic activity in the area of operation or trauma.

The programme of investigation, first served as basic research and was then directed towards the clinical situation for recording the partly contradictory or still unknown haemostasis values in the CSF. This necessitated that the immunochemical, enzymatic, enzymatic-fluorometric, biophysical and chromogenic substrate methods should be adapted to low quantities of protein for the quantitative determination of activators, inhibitors, zymogens, enzymes, the fibrin substrate and its degradation products.

The results obtained with the prospective series of tests applying selective methods with objective data recording confirm the operating hypothesis that, on principle, a distinction must be made between the proteins of normal CSF in cases of intact BBB and the pathological protein patterns, not typical of CSF, caused by disturbances of permeation. The CSF space, therefore, must be regarded as a compartment largely insulated by the BBB. That is why the unqualified interpretation is wrong, when it states that the CSF, in general, shows a fibrinolytic activity, no matter whether the CSF is formed under physiological or pathological conditions, or whether it represents a mixture of blood and CSF.

CSF formed when the BBB is normal has no fibrinolytic activity. The plasminogen activator antigen always present in CSF does not become effective because the quantity of plasminogen in CSF is well below normal for the measurable fibrinolytic activity. In the case of diseases accompanied by disturbance of the BBB, the proteins of the fibrinolytic system in the CSF increasingly penetrate in proportion to the disturbance of BBB, and thus enable the CSF to some extent to become a fibrinolytically active fluid. A temporarily limited breakdown of the BBB in the case of bleeding into the CSF space permits the unhampered transfer of all the factors required for the fibrinolytic system, as well as the inhibitors. Due to the dilution of blood by CSF no interaction between the inhibitors and plasmin will occur, so that a free fibrinolytic activity exists at all times. Hence, the plasmin activity of CSF is no more than a function of the BBB disturbance. With the plasmin-catalysed fibrin degradation to FDP always taking place in blood-stained CSF in vivo, it thus becomes possible for the clinician to make the important diagnostic distinction between artificial blood contamination and an autochthonous SAH. The results obtained also confirm a coagulation-promoting effect of the CSF, rich in thromboplastin, in connection with blood, so that the old ideas, stating that the blood in the CSF is not capable of clotting, must be revised for good.

The permeation of the coagulation and fibrinolytic inhibitors also largely correlates with the degree of disturbance of the BBB. The regularity of the existing "restricted diffusion" was again substantiated by the immunochemical demonstration for the first time of antithrombin III, α_2 antiplasmin and C-1 esterase inhibitor in the CSF. In the event that a cerebrogenesis is out of the question, increase in α_1 antitrypsin and α_2 macroglobulin must be considered as sensitive indicators of BBB disturbance (influx syndrome).

The second part of this study consists of a basic concept of all significant reactions in the ruptured aneurysm with emphasis on the haemostatic functions, including wound healing. Follow-up of coagulation values in the blood after SAH showed changes in the extrinsic and intrinsic pathway, which need to be compensated therapeutically. The results obtained in analyses justify the administration of vitamin K_1, because all healing of wounds, cerebral vascular lesions included, presupposes optimum values of coagulation factors in order to prevent rebleeding due to a bleeding tendency caused by a factor deficiency. There were no indications of disseminated intravascular coagulation in SAH and recurrent SAH patients.

With the rise in the incidence of recurrent SAH which is accompanied by such an unfavourable prognosis, the influencing of fibrinolysis by drugs represents another important problem, that could be solved by chemical control on the basis of pharmacokinetic observations. The good results obtained by oral and parenteral AFT with EACA and AMCA demonstrates that aneurysmal rebleedings are, in the main, due to inadequate clot formation on the tissue lesion at the site of rupture or due to increased physiological fibrinolysis in the granulation- and connective-tissue during the phases of proliferation.

The concentrations of antifibrinolytic drugs in the CSF established at present also indicate that the required concentration for the inhibition of fibrinolysis is not attained despite a disturbed BBB, so that it is not possible to achieve optimum inhibition of local fibrinolytic activity around the vascular lesion and in the CSF, notwithstanding the fact that the doses were high. On the assumption that the basic concept of AFT is correct, inhibition of local fibrinolysis is just a matter of the concentration of the antifibrinolytic drugs at the site of action, disregarding other possible factors which might contribute to bleeding, with no relationship to the haemostatic system.

In spite of high oral and parenteral PAMBA dosage in SAH patients and in those with a disturbed BBB, it was only possible to attain concentrations of PAMBA in the CSF which were well below the limit of effectiveness. After preceding animal experiments in which favourable results regarding the concentration and half-life of PAMBA in CSF were obtained, intrathecal AFT with PAMBA was used as an alternative to oral and parenteral AFT with EACA and AMCA.

Because of possible complications in SAH patients the dose of intrathecal PAMBA initially instilled was comparatively low. Subsequently, doses were given which would produce a level in the CSF 20 times the effective concentration required for fibrinolysis inhibition. The CSF withdrawn under strict clinical indications permits the determination of half-life and the results confirm full inhibition of the fibrinolytic reaction in the CSF up to 36 hours after intrathecal AFT, using 50 mg of PAMBA. The absence of side-effects and the in vitro results which show that no biotransformation of PAMBA in CSF takes place, as well as the high degree of diffusion into a fibrin clot are additional criteria which favour the concept of this route of administration.

According to the present state of knowledge AFT with high doses of oral and parenteral EACA and AMCA is likewise confirmed as prophylaxis of recurrent bleeding after SAH, as is shown by good clinical results, although the drug concentration in the CSF evidently does not reach optimum values.

Compared with this it is possible to ensure continuously the necessary concentration by intrathecal instillation of low doses of PAMBA in combination with similarly low intravenous doses. This is done to inhibit completely the exogenic and/or endogenic fibrinolysis working on the thrombotically occluded aneurysm. Such an intrathecal AFT with PAMBA, administered for maximum 12 days and showing no side-effects, represents a reasonable risk that should be accepted by the SAH patient. This statement is substantiated by CT scan controls. Cerebral and/or peripheral thrombotic complications can be ruled out and have not been observed.

AFT should always be carried out pre-operatively in cases of bleeding from a source that cannot be verified angiographically, and also in such cases which do not allow an operation. Vascular surgery demands priority at all times because although a thrombosed aneurysm with subsequent fibrous organization represents an occlusion it will always remain a *locus minoris resistentiae.*

References

1. Adams, H. P., Current status of antifibrinolytic therapy for treatment of patients with aneurysmal subarachnoid hemorrhage. Stroke *13* (1982), 256—263.
2. Adams, H. P., Nibbelink, D. W., Torner, J. C., Sahs, A. L., Antifibrinolytic therapy in patients with aneurysmal subarachnoid hemorrhage. A report of the cooperative aneurysm study. Arch. Neurol. *38* (1981), 25—29.
3. Adler, H., Untersuchungen zur Pathogenese des zerebralen Vasospasmus. Neurochirurgia (Stuttg.) *17* (1974), 202—208.
4. Albrechtsen, O. K., Storm, O., Classen, M., Fibrinolytic activity in some human body fluids. Scand. J. Clin. Lab. Invest. *10* (1958), 310—318.
5. Alvarez-Garijo, J. A., Vilchez, J. J., Aznar, J. A., Preoperative treatment of ruptured intracranial aneurysms with tranexamic acid and monitoring of fibrinolytic activity. J. Neurosurg. *52* (1980), 453—455.
6. Ambrus, C. M., Marcus, G., Plasmin-antiplasmin complex as a reservoir of fibrinolytic enzymes. Am. J. Physiol. *199* (1960), 491—494.
7. Ameen, A. A., Illingworth, R., Anti-fibrinolytic treatment in the pre-operative management of subarachnoid haemorrhage caused by ruptured intracranial aneurysm. J. Neurol. Neurosurg. Psychiatry *44* (1981), 220—226.
8. Anderson, M., Matthews, K. B., Stuart, J., Coagulation and fibrinolytic activity of cerebrospinal fluid. J. Clin. Pathol. *31* (1978), 488—492.
9. Andersson, L., Nilsson, I. M., Liedberg, G., Nilsson, L., Rybo, G., Eriksson, O., Granstrand, B., Melander, B., Vergleichende Untersuchungen von trans-4-(Aminomethyl)-cyclohexancarbonsäure, Aminocapronsäure und p-Aminomethylbenzoesäure. Arzneimittelforsch. *21* (1971), 424—429.
10. Astedt, B., Liedholm, P., Tranexamic acid and fibrinolytic activity of the vessel wall. Experientia *30* (1974), 776—777.
11. Astedt, B., Liedholm, P., Wingerup, L., The effect of tranexamic acid on the fibrinolytic activity of vein walls. Ann. Chir. Gynaecol. *67* (1978), 203—205.
12. Astedt, B., Pandolfi, M., On release and synthesis of fibrinolytic activators in human organ culture. Rev. Eur. Etudes Clin. et Biol. *17* (1972), 261—267.
13. Astrup, T., Tissue activators of plasminogen. Fed. Proc. *25* (1966), 42—51.
14. Astrup, T., Fibrinolysis: An overview. In: Progress in Chemical Fibrinolysis and Thrombolysis (Davidson, J. F., Rowan, M. R., Samama, M. M., Desnoyers, P. C., eds.), Vol. 3, pp. 1—57. New York: Raven Press. 1978.
15. Astrup, T., Fibrinolytic activity in the brain and its membranes. In: Cerebrum, Blutgerinnung und Hämostase (Marx, R., Thies, H. A., Hrsg.), pp. 53—58. XXII. Hamburger Symposium über Blutgerinnung 1979. Wissenschaftlicher Dienst Roche. 1980.

16. Auer, L., Wendt, P., Huber, P., Blümel, G., Untersuchungen über proteolytische Enzymaktivität nach experimentellem Schädel-Hirn-Trauma. In: Neue Aspekte der Trasylol Therapie (Breddin, K., Eisenbach, J., Haberland, G. L., Schnells, G., Hrsg.), Vol. 7, pp. 229—239. Stuttgart: F. K. Schattauer. 1974.
17. Bachmann, J., Untersuchungen der Blutgerinnung nach Commotio cerebri. Medizinische Dissertation. Heidelberg 1977.
18. Bang, N. U., Beller, F. K., Deutsch, E., Mammen, E. F., (eds.), Thrombosis and bleeding disorders. Theory and methods. Stuttgart: G. Thieme. New York-London: Academic Press. 1971.
19. Barnhardt, M. I., Riddle, J. M., Cellular localization of profibrinolysin (plasminogen). Blood *21* (1963), 306—321.
20. Beck, O. J., Preoperative treatment of intracranial aneurysms. In: Cerebral Aneurysms. Advances in Diagnosis and Therapy (Pia, H. W., Langmaid, C., Zierski, J., eds.), pp. 197—200. Berlin-Heidelberg-New York: Springer. 1979.
21. Beck, O. J., Marx, R., Konservative Therapie der Subarachnoidal- und Aneurysmablutung. In: Cerebrum, Blutgerinnung und Hämostase (Marx, R., Thies, H. A., Hrsg.), pp. 159—164. XXII. Hamburger Symposium über Blutgerinnung. 1979. Wissenschaftlicher Dienst Roche. 1980.
22. Beck, O. J., Wieser, H. X., Die Bedeutung des Vasospasmus für die Prognose nach Aneurysmablutung. Zentralbl. Neurochir. *35* (1974), 21—34.
23. Beneke, G., Der Thrombus als pathologisch anatomisches Substrat. Thromb. Diath. Haemorrh. Suppl. *32* (1969), 217—239.
24. Bennett, M., Sills, J. A., Cerebral haemorrhage in haemophilia. Postgrad. Med. J. *54* (1978), 628.
25. Bewermeyer, H., Szelies, B., Lumenta, C., Heiss, W. D., Änderungen im Verlauf nach spontanen Subarachnoidalblutungen aus neurologischer Sicht. Fortschr. Neurol. Psychiatr. *50* (1982), 247—257.
26. Biggs, R. (ed.), Human blood coagulation, haemostasis and thrombosis. Oxford: Blackwell sci. publ. 1972.
27. Bohm, E., Hugosson, R., Results of surgical treatment of 200 consecutive cerebral arterial aneurysms. Acta Neurol. Scand. *46* (1970), 43—52.
28. Borchardt, U., Siedschlag, W. D., Die Bedeutung des EEG für die Bestimmung des Angiographie- und Operationstermines bei Subarachnoidalblutung nach Aneurysmaruptur. Zentralbl. Neurochir. *41* (1980), 303—310.
29. Botterell, E. H., Lougheed, W. M., Scott, J. W., Vandewater, S. L., Hyperthermia and interruption of carotid, or carotid and vertebral circulation in the surgical management of intracranial aneurysms. J. Neurosurg. *13* (1956), 1—42.
30. Brueton, M. J., Tugwell, P., Whittle, H. C., Greenood, B. M., Fibrin degradation products in the serum and cerebrospinal fluid of patients with group A meningococcal meningitis. J. Clin. Pathol. *27* (1974), 402—404.
31. Burchiel, K. J., Schmer, G., A method for monitoring antifibrinolytic therapy in patients with ruptured intracranial aneurysms. J. Neurosurg. *54* (1981), 12—15.

32. Cervos-Navarro, J., Betz, E., Matakas, F., Wüllenweber, R. (eds.), The cerebral vessel wall. New York: Raven Press. 1975.
33. Chandra, B., Treatment of subarachnoid hemorrhage from ruptured intracranial aneurysm with tranexamic acid. A double blind clinical trial. Ann. Neurol. *3* (1978), 502—504.
34. Chesterman, C. N., Allington, M. J., Sharp, A. A., Relationship of plasminogen activator to fibrin. Nature, New Biol. *238* (1972), 15—17.
35. Chowdhary, U. M., Carey, P. C., Hussein, M. M., Prevention of early recurrence of spontaneous subarachnoid haemorrhage by ε-aminocaproic acid. Lancet *I* (1979), 741—743.
36. Clark, J. A., Finelli, R. E., Netsky, M. G., Disseminated intravascular coagulation following cranial trauma—case report. J. Neurosurg. *52* (1980), 266—275.
37. Clendenon, N. R., Allen, N., Komatsu, T., Liss, L., Gordon, W. A., Heimberger, K., Biochemical alterations in the anoxic-ischemic lesion of rat brain. Arch. Neurol. *25* (1971), 432—448.
38. Collen, D., Wiman, B., Fast-acting plasmin inhibitor in human plasma. Blood *51* (1978), 563—569.
39. Copley, A. L., Roles of platelets in physiological defense mechanisms and pathological conditions. Folia Haematol. (Leipz.) *106* (1979), 732—764.
40. Corkill, G., Earlier operation and antifibrinolytic therapy in the management of aneurysmal subarachnoid haemorrhage. Med. J. Aus. *1* (1974), 468—470.
41. Corkill, G., Epsilon-aminocaproic acid and subarachnoid haemorrhage. (Letter) Lancet *II* (1974), 1319.
42. Crompton, M. R., Mechanism of growth and rupture in cerebral berry aneurysms. Brit. Med. J. *1* (1966), 1138—1142.
43. Davidson, J. F. (ed.), Fibrinolysis and its inhibition. J. Clin. Pathol. *33*, Suppl. *14* (1980), 1—80.
44. Davidson, J. F., Samama, M. M., Desnoyers, P. C. (eds.), Progress in Chemical Fibrinolysis and Thrombolysis, Vol. *2*. New York: Raven Press. 1976.
45. Davies, D., Howell, D. A., Tranexamic acid and arterial thrombosis. (Letter) Lancet *I* (1977), 49.
46. Deutsch, E., Blutgerinnung und Operation. München-Berlin-Wien: Urban und Schwarzenberg. 1973.
47. Dommasch, D., Mertens, H. G. (eds.), Cerebrospinalflüssigkeit CSF. Stuttgart-New York: G. Thieme. 1980.
48. Dube, R. K., Dube, B., Ahmad, M., Saha, P. K., Rao, P. V. B., Katiyar, B. C., Presence of complete plasminogen activator in the cerebrospinal fluid. Indian J. Med. Res. *69* (1979), 474—475.
49. Dube, R. K., Saha, P. K., Dube, B., Katiyar, B. C., Rao, P. V. B., Fibrinogen, fibrinogen degradation products and fibrinolytic activity in cerebrospinal fluid in stroke. Indian J. Med. Res. *72* (1980), 454—458.
50. Ebhardt, G., Wüllenweber, R., Cervos-Navarro, J., The ultrastructure of the aneurysmatic vessel wall. In: The Cerebral Vessel Wall (Cervos-Navarro, J.,

Betz, E., Matakas, F., Wüllenweber, R., eds.), pp. 67—74. New York: Raven Press. 1976.

51. Endler, S., Intrakranielle Blutungen. Ärztl. Fortbild. Jena *7* (1973), 341—342.
52. Erdös, E. G. (ed.), Bradykinin Kallidin and Kallikrein. Handbook of Experimental Pharmacology, Vol. *25*. Berlin-Heidelberg-New York: Springer. 1970.
53. Ettinger, M. G., Coagulation abnormalities in subarachnoid hemorrhage. Stroke *1* (1970), 139—142.
54. Ewald, T., Mahaley, S., Goodrich, J., Wilkinson, R., Silver, D., Experimental epsilon-aminocaproic acid (EACA) administration in the presence of subarachnoid blood. J. Neurosurg. *35* (1971), 657—663.
55. Fareed, J., Messmore, H. L., Fenton, J. W., Brinkhous, K. M. (eds.), Perspectives in Hemostasis. New York-Oxford-Toronto-Sydney-Paris-Frankfurt: Pergamon Press. 1981.
56. Farina, M. L., Levati, A., Paino, R., Myocardial infarction during antifibrinolytic treatment of subarachnoid haemorrhage. Thromb. Haemost. *42* (1979), 1347—1348.
57. Felgenhauer, K., Vergleichende Disk-Elektrophorese von Serum und Liquor cerebrospinalis. Stuttgart: G. Thieme. 1971.
58. Felgenhauer, K., Protein size and cerebrospinal fluid composition. Klin. Wochenschr. *52* (1974), 1158—1164.
59. Filizzolo, F., Angelo, V. D., Collice, M., Ferrara, M., Donati, M. B., Porta, M., Fibrinolytic activity in blood and cerebrospinal fluid in subarachnoid hemorrhage from ruptured intracranial saccular aneurysm before and during EACA treatment. Eur. Neurol. *17* (1978), 43—47.
60. Flamm, E. S., Ransohoff, J., Preoperative management of ruptured intracranial aneurysms with antifibrinolytic treatment. In: Cerebral Aneurysms. Advances in Diagnosis and Therapy (Pia, H. W., Langmaid, C., Zierski, J., eds.), pp. 200—202. Berlin-Heidelberg-New York: Springer. 1979.
61. Fleischer, A. S., Tindall, G. T., Cerebral vasospasm following aneurysm rupture. J. Neurosurg. *52* (1980), 149—152.
62. Fletcher, A. P., Alkjaersig, N., The role of thrombosis in cerebrovascular occlusive disease. In: Venous and Arterial Thrombosis (Joist, J. H., Sherman, L. A., eds.). New York-San Francisco-London: Grune & Stratton Inc. 1979.
63. Fodstad, H., Tranexamic acid (AMCA) in aneurysmal subarachnoid haemorrhage. J. Clin. Pathol. *33*, Suppl. *14* (1980), 68—73.
64. Fodstad, H., Tranexamic acid as therapeutic agents in aneurysmal subarachnoid haemorrhage. Clinical, laboratory and experimental studies. Umea University Medical Dissertations. New Series No. 60. 1980.
65. Fodstad, H., Antifibrinolytic treatment in subarachnoid haemorrhage. Present state. Acta Neurochir. (Wien) *63* (1982), 233—244.
66. Fodstad, H., Forssell, A., Liliequist, B., Schannong, M., Antifibrinolysis with tranexamic acid in aneurysmal subarachnoid hemorrhage. A consecutive controlled clinical trial. Neurosurgery *8* (1981), 158—165.

67. Fodstad, H., Forssell, A., Liliequist, B., Schannong, M., West, K. A., Antifibrinolytics and subarachnoid haemorrhage: Results from two controlled clinical trials using tranexamic acid (AMCHA). Acta Neurochir. (Wien) *51* (1979), 131.
68. Fodstad, H., Kok, P., Algers, G., Fibrinolytic activity (FA) of cerebral tissue after experimental subarachnoid haemorrhage (SAH). Effect of tranexamic acid (AMCA). In: Synthetic Fibrinolytic Thrombolytic Agents. Progress in Fibrinolysis. Fifth international conference Malmö, Sweden 1980. Abstract book 59.
69. Fodstad, H., Liliequist, B., Spontaneous thrombosis of ruptured intracranial aneurysms during treatment with tranexamic acid (AMCA) report of three cases. Acta Neurochir. (Wien) *49* (1979), 129—144.
70. Fodstad, H., Liliequist, B., Schannong, M., Thulin, C., Tranexamic acid in the preoperative management of ruptured intracranial aneurysms. Surg. Neurol. *9* (1978), 9—15.
71. Fodstad, H., Nilsson, I. M., Coagulation and fibrinolysis in blood and cerebrospinal fluid after aneurysmal subarachnoid haemorrhage: Effect of tranexamic acid (AMCA). Acta Neurochir. (Wien) *56* (1981), 25—38.
72. Fodstad, H., Pilbrant, A., Schannong, M., Strömberg, S., Determination of tranexamic acid (AMCA) and fibrin/fibrinogen degradation products in cerebrospinal fluid after aneurysmal subarachnoid haemorrhage. Acta Neurochir. (Wien) *58* (1981), 1—13.
73. Fodstad, H., Thulin, C. A., Concerning the paper written by Gelmers, H. J.: Management of patients with subarachnoid haemorrhage with tranexamic acid. Gelmers, H. J.: Reply to the letter of Fodstad, H. and Thulin, C. A. Acta Neurochir. (Wien) *54* (1980), 127—131.
74. Fortuna, L. A., Prieto-Valiente, L., Long-term prognosis in surgically treated intracranial aneurysms. Part I; Mortality. J. Neurosurg. *54* (1981), 26—34.
75. Friemel, H. (Hrsg.), Immunologische Arbeitsmethoden. Jena: G. Fischer. 1976.
76. Fujii, T., Increased fibrinolysis of cerebrospinal fluid in dogs with the intracranial paraffin clot. J. Physiol. Soc. Jap. *32* (1970), 265—274.
77. Fujii, S., Moriya, H., Suzuki, T., Kinins—II B, Systemic proteases and cellular function. New York: Plenum publ. corp. 1979.
78. Gänshirt, H. (Hrsg.), Der Hirnkreislauf. Stuttgart: G. Thieme. 1972.
79. Gaffney, P. J., Balkuv-Ulutin, S. (eds.), Fibrinolysis. London-New York-San Francisco: Academic Press. 1978.
80. Gelmers, H. J., Prevention of recurrence of spontaneous subarachnoid haemorrhage by tranexamic acid. Acta Neurochir. (Wien) *52* (1980), 45—50.
81. Gelmers, H. J., Beks, J. W. F., Journee, H. L., Regional cerebral blood flow in patients with subarachnoid haemorrhage. Acta Neurochir. (Wien) *47* (1979), 245—251.
82. Gibbs, J. R., Corkill, A. G. L., Use of an antifibrinolytic agent (tranexamic acid) in the management of ruptured intracranial aneurysms. Postgrad. Med. J. *47* (1971), 199—200.

83. Gibbs, J. R., Gorman, P. O., Fibrinolysis in subarachnoid haemorrhage. Postgrad. Med. J. *43* (1967), 779—784.

84. Girvin, J. P., The use antifibrinolytic agents in the preoperative treatment of ruptured intracranial aneurysms. Trans. Am. Neurol. Assoc. *98* (1973), 150—152.

85. Glasner, H., Piepgras, U., CSF circulation and blood-CSF barrier. Eur. Neurol. *17* (1978), 280—285.

86. Glick, R., Green, D., Tsào, C., Witt, W. A., Yu, A. T. W., Raimondi, A. J., High dose aminocaproic acid prolongs the bleeding time and increases rebleeding and intraoperative hemorrhage in patients with subarachnoid hemorrhage. Neurosurgery *9* (1981), 398—401.

87. Gonsette, R., Incidence clinique des troubles de la perméabilité capillaire cérébrale (barrière hématoencéphalique). Paris: Masson et Cie. 1972.

88. Grote, E., Walther, C., Wenker, H., Protrahierte Hirnmassenblutung bei hyperfibrinolytischer Hypofibrinogenämie. Nervenarzt *40* (1969), 385—389.

89. Halse, T., Bedeutung und Reaktionskinetik der Defibrinierung in den serösen Körperhöhlen. Schweiz. Med. Wochenschr. *79* (1949), 388.

90. Hamer, J., Häufigkeit und klinische Bedeutung des cerebralen Vasospasmus nach aneurysmatischer Subarachnoidalblutung. Nervenarzt *52* (1981), 108—113.

91. Hassler, O., Morphological studies on the large cerebral arteries with a reference to the aetiology of subarachnoid haemorrhage. Acta Psychiat. Neurol. Scand. Suppl. 154, *36* (1961), 1—145.

92. Hassler, O., Fodstad, H., Fibrinolytic activity in the walls of cerebral saccular aneurysms. Acta Neurochir. (Wien) *37* (1977), 49—55.

93. Hedlund, P. O., Postoperative venous thrombosis in benign prostatic disease. Scand. J. Urol. Nephrol. Suppl. *27* (1975), 46—53.

94. Heidrich, R., Die subarachnoideale Blutung. Leipzig: G. Thieme. 1970.

95. Heidrich, R., Subarachnoid haemorrhage. In: Handbook Clinical Neurology (Vinken, P. J., Bruyn, G. W., eds.), *12/II*, pp. 68—204. Amsterdam: North-Holland publ. company. 1972.

96. Heidrich, R., Hindersin, P., Endler, S., Zur Bedeutung der intrathekalen antifibrinolytischen Therapie von Subarachnoidalblutungen mit p-Aminomethylbenzoesäure. Dtsch. Gesundh.-Wesen *34* (1979), 1553—1554.

97. Heidrich, R., Markwardt, F., Endler, S., Hindersin, P., Antifibrinolytic therapy of subarachnoid hemorrhage by intrathecal administration of p-aminomethylbenzoic acid. J. Neurol. *219* (1978), 83—85.

98. Heimburger, N., Karges, H. E., Immunologische Gerinnungsdiagnostik. Laboratoriumsblätter für die medizinische Diagnostik — Behring. *26* (1976), 45—60.

99. Hellinger, J., Vogel, G., Untersuchungen über die fibrinolytische Aktivität des Liquor cerebrospinalis und ihre Beeinflußbarkeit durch PAMBA. Folia Haematol. (Leipz.) *87* (1967), 61—65.

100. Hemmer, R., Komplikationen beim atrio-ventrikulären Shunt und ihre Vermeidung. Z. Kinderchir. *5* (1967), 10—24.

101. Hemmer, R., Schneider, J., Maleknasri, F., Zur Frage der fibrinolytischen Wirksamkeit des Liquors. Nervenarzt *6* (1970), 303—305.
102. Hernándes-Richter, H. J., Struck, H., Die Wundheilung. Theoretische und praktische Grundlagen. Stuttgart: G. Thieme. 1970.
103. Herschlein, J. K., Steichele, D. F., Die Wirkung des Fibrinolyseinhibitors AMCHA auf die Blutgerinnung bei gesteigerter thromboplastischer Aktivität. Klin. Wochenschr. *46* (1968), 102—106.
104. Hindersin, P., Immunologische Gerinnungs- und Fibrinolysediagnostik unter Berücksichtigung von Intermediärprodukten. Z. Med. Lab.-Diagn. *20* (1979), 136—141.
105. Hindersin, P., Das Gerinnungs- und Fibrinolyse-Enzymsystem im Liquor cerebrospinalis unter normaler und gestörter Blut-Hirn-Schrankenfunktion bei intrakraniellen Blutungen und deren biochemische Beeinflussung. Jena: Wiss. B-Dissertation (degree of habilitation) Sect. Math.-Naturw. 1981.
106. Hindersin, P., Unpublished results. 1983.
107. Hindersin, P., Endler, S., In vitro Versuche zur Bestimmung der Gerinnungsaktivität in normalen, entzündlich veränderten und blutigen Liquores. Folia Haematol. (Leipzig) *107* (1980), 919—927.
108. Hindersin, P., Endler, S., Heidrich, R., Gerinnungsphysiologische Verlaufskontrollen bei Subarachnoidealblutungen und deren therapeutische Konsequenzen. Psychiatr. Neurol. Med. Psychol. (Leipzig) *34* (1982), 236—241.
109. Hindersin, P., Endler, S., Sedlarik, K., Tierexperimentelle Untersuchungen zur Pharmakokinetik von p-Aminomethylbenzoesäure (PAMBA) im Liquor nach intrathekaler Applikation. Folia Haematol. (Leipzig) *106* (1979), 619—625.
110. Hindersin, P., Heidrich, R., Hämostatische Abläufe bei Aneurysmablutungen. Psychiatr. Neurol. Med. Psychol. (Leipzig) *29* (1977), 129—144.
111. Hindersin, P., Heidrich, R., In vitro Versuche zur Klärung der fibrinolytischen Aktivität im Normalliquor. Psychiatr. Neurol. Med. Psychol. (Leipzig) *29* (1977), 275—284.
112. Hindersin, P., Heidrich, R., In vitro Versuche zur Klärung der fibrinolytischen Aktivität in entzündlich veränderten und blutigen Liquores mit pathologischen Proteinwerten. Psychiatr. Neurol. Med. Psychol. (Leipzig) *29* (1977), 465—473.
113. Hindersin, P., Heidrich, R., Die Fibrin(ogen)-Spaltprodukte(FSP)-Konzentration als diagnostischer Parameter zur Unterscheidung von artifiziell und essentiell blutigen Liquores. Psychiatr. Neurol. Med. Psychol. (Leipzig) *30* (1978), 36—39.
114. Hindersin, P., Heidrich, R., Thrombelastographische und immunologische Fibrinolyse-Bestimmungen in entzündlich veränderten und artifiziell blutigen Liquores unter Verwendung von Fibrin(ogen)-Substrat. Psychiatr. Neurol. Med. Psychol. (Leipzig) *31* (1979), 197—201.
115. Hindersin, P., Heidrich, R., Fibrinolytische Inhibitorproteine des hämostaseologischen Systems in normalen, entzündlich veränderten und blutigen Liquores. Psychiatr. Neurol. Med. Psychol. (Leipzig) *32* (1980), 328—337.

116. Hindersin, P., Heidrich, R., Endler, S., Beitrag zur antifibrinolytischen Therapie bei Subarachnoidealblutungen. Untersuchungen über die Permeation der oral applizierten para-Aminomethylbenzoesäure in den Liquor. Psychiatr. Neurol. Med. Psychol. (Leipzig) *32* (1980), 214—219.

117. Hindersin, P., Körting, H. J., Voss, G. R., Microscope fluorometry as a micro-technique for recording fibrinolytic plasma activities. Jena review. *19* (1974), 216—217.

118. Hindersin, P., Richter, M., Senf, L., Endler, S., Experimentelle Untersuchungen zur Diffusion von Antifibrinolytika in Fibrinabscheidungsthromben. Ein Beitrag zur intrathekalen antifibrinolytischen Therapie bei Subarachnoidealblutungen. Folia Haematol. (Leipzig) *109* (1982), 313—318.

119. Hindersin, P., Zwiener, U., Körting, H. J., Eine mikroskopfluoreszenzphotometrische Methode zur quantitativen Bestimmung der fibrinolytischen Aktivität in kleinen Blutmengen. Haematologia (Budapest) *6* (1972), 459—466.

120. Hoffmann, E. P., Koo, A. H., Cerebral thrombosis associated with Amicar therapy. Radiology *131* (1979), 687—689.

121. Huhn, A., Die Thrombosen der intrakraniellen Venen und Sinus. Stuttgart: Schattauer. 1965.

122. Hunt, W. E., Hess, R. M., Surgical risk as related to time of intervention in the repair of intracranial aneurysms. J. Neurosurg. *28* (1968), 14—19.

123. Hunter, R., Thomson, T., Reynolds, C. M., Pitcher, P. M., Fibrin/fibrinogen degradation products in cerebrospinal fluid of patients admitted to a psychiatric unit. J. Neurol. Neurosurg. Psychiatry *37* (1974), 249—251.

124. Imanaga, H., Osugi, T., Kagawa, M., Kitamura, K., Fibrinolytic activity of cerebrospinal fluid in subarachnoid hemorrhage. Neurol. Surg. (Japan) *5* (1977), 51—58.

125. Ishii, M., Suzuki, S., Iwabuchi, T., Julow, J., Effect of antifibrinolytic therapy on subarachnoid fibrosis in dogs after experimental subarachnoid haemorrhage. Acta Neurochir. (Wien) *54* (1980), 17—24.

126. Ito, H., Komai, T., Yamamoto, S., Fibrinolytic enzyme in the lining walls of chronic subdural hematoma. J. Neurosurg. *48* (1978), 197—201.

127. Jatkowitz, S., Epsilon-aminocaproic acid and possible pulmonary emboli. N. Engl. J. Med. *290* (1974), 861.

128. Julow, J., Prevention of subarachnoid fibrosis after subarachnoid haemorrhage with urokinase. Acta Neurochir. (Wien) *51* (1979), 53—61.

129. Kagström, E., Palma, L., Influence of antifibrinolytic treatment on the morbidity in patients with subarachnoid haemorrhage. Acta Neurol. Scand. *48* (1977), 257—258.

130. Kaller, H., Pharmakologie des Trasylols. In: Neue Aspekte der Trasylol Therapie (Marx, R., Imdahl, H., Haberland, G. L., Hrsg.) *2*, pp. 11—17. Stuttgart: F. K. Schattauer. 1968.

131. Kappert, H., Experimentelle und klinische Untersuchungen über die arterielle Thrombogenese und Fibrinolyse. Basel-Stuttgart: Schwabe. 1962.

132. Karges, H. E., Schwinn, H., Becker, U., Heimburger, N., (eds.), Großer

Gerinnungsstatus — Gerinnungsdiagnostik in Klinik, Labor und Praxis. Behringwerke AG Medizinische Information und Vertrieb 1979.

133. Karris, R., Concerning the paper written by Ramirez-Lassepas, M., Antifibrinolytic therapy in subarachnoid hemorrhage caused by ruptured intracranial aneurysm. Ramirez-Lassepas, M., Reply to the letter of Karris, R., Neurology (N.Y.) *31* (1981), 1498—1499.

134. Kassell, N. F., Torner, J. C., The international cooperative study on timing of aneurysm surgery. Acta Neurochir. (Wien) *63* (1982), 119—123.

135. Kaste, M., Ramsay, M., Effect of tranexamic acid on fatal rebleeds after subarachnoid haemorrhage. Double-blind study. Acta Neurol. Scand. *57* (1978), Suppl. 67, 254.

136. Kaste, M., Ramsay, M., Antifibrinolytic treatment of patients with subarachnoid haemorrhage. Acta Neurochir. (Wien) *51* (1979), 131.

137. Kaste, M., Ramsay, M., Tranexamic acid in subarachnoid hemorrhage: A double-blind study. Stroke *10* (1979), 519—522.

138. Kaste, M., Troupp, H., Subarachnoid haemorrhage: Long term follow-up results of late surgical versus conservative treatment. Brit. Med. J. *1* (1978), 1310—1311.

139. von Kaulla, K. N., Ostendorf, P., von Kaulla, E., Beobachtungen über die Wirkung von Angiogrammen und Pneumenzephalogrammen auf Parameter der Gerinnung und Fibrinolyse. Thromb. Diath. Haemorrh. Suppl. *58* (1974), 257—271.

140. Kleine, T. O. (Hrsg.), Neue Labormethoden für die Liquordiagnostik. Stuttgart-New York: G. Thieme. 1980.

141. Klöcking, H. P., Zum Mechanismus der Thrombolyse durch Streptokinase. Folia Haematol. (Leipzig) *106* (1979), 885—898.

142. Kölmel, H. W., Die intrathekale Gabe von Zytostatika. Nervenarzt *49* (1978), 685—696.

143. Kobayashi, S., Sugita, K., Tanizaki, Y., Nakagawa, F., Takemae, T., Mortality study of patients with subarachnoid haemorrhage at university hospitals and their affiliated hospitals in Japan. Acta Neurochir. (Wien) *63* (1982), 175—183.

144. Koos, W. T., Perneczky, A., Timing of surgery for ruptured aneurysms—experience from 800 consecutive cases. Acta Neurochir. (Wien) *63* (1982), 125—133.

145. Kovalainen, S., Myllylä, V. V., Tolonen, U., Hokkanen, E., Recurrent subarachnoid haemorrhages in patient with Hageman factor deficiency. (Letter) Lancet *I* (1979), 1035—1036.

146. Kröss, R., Barolin, G. S., Die Subarachnoidalblutung aus konservativ-neurologischer Sicht. In: Die zerebrale Apoplexie (Barolin, G. S., Hrsg.). Stuttgart: Enke. 1980.

147. Kruithof, E. K., Bachmann, F., Studies on the binding of tissue plasminogen activator to fibrinogen and fibrin. In: Fibrinogen (Henschen, A., Graeff, H., Lottspeich, F., eds.), pp. 377—387. Berlin-New York: De Gruyter. 1982.

148. Kuhn, W., Graeff, H., Gerinnungsstörungen in der Geburtshilfe. Stuttgart: G. Thieme. 1970.

149. Kwaan, H. C., Astrup, T., Fibrinolytic activity of reparative connective tissue. J. Pathol. Bact. *87* (1964), 409—414.

150. Kwaan, H. C., Astrup, T., Fibrinolytic activity of vascular endothelium. Thromb. Diath. Haemorrh. *18* (1967), 296—297.

151. Kwaan, H. C., McFadzean, J. S., On plasma fibrinolytic activity induced by ischaemia. Clin. Sci. *15* (1956), 245—257.

152. Labadie, E. L., Glover, D., Local alterations of hemostatic-fibrinolytic mechanisms in reforming subdural hematomas. Neurology (N.Y.) *25* (1975), 669—675.

153. Lajtha, A., Ford, D. H., Brain barrier systems. Progress in Brain Res. *29*, Amsterdam-London-New York: Elsevier. 1968.

154. Laki, K. (ed.), Fibrinogen. New York: Marcel Dekker Inc. 1968.

155. Laurell, C. B., Electro-immuno-assay. Scand. J. Clin. Lab. Invest. *29* Suppl. 124 (1972), 21—37.

156. Leska, P., Krupka, J., Intratekální aplikace antifibrinolytik u subarachnoidálního krvácení. Cesk. Neurol. Neurochir. *46* (1983), 411—412.

157. Levati, A., Minella, C., Farina, M. L., Dangelo, V., Potential hazards of antifibrinolytic treatment in subarachnoid haemorrhage. Thromb. Haemost. *44* (1980), 170.

158. Levi, B. J., Silver, D., Treatment of subarachnoid hemorrhage: The ability of epsilon-aminocaproic acid to cross the blood brain barrier and reduce the spinal fluid fibrinolytic activity. Surg. Forum *19* (1968), 413—414.

159. Lindner, J., Huber, P., Biochemie und morphologische Grundlagen der Wundheilung und ihre Beeinflussung. Med. Welt *24* (1973), 897—911.

160. Lindsay, K. W., Volo, G., Teasdale, G. M., Concerning the paper written by Adams, H. P., *et al.*: Antifibrinolytic therapy in subarachnoid hemorrhage. Adams, H. P., Kassell, N. F., Torner, J. C., Sahs, A. L.: Reply to the letter of Lindsay, K. W., *et al.* J. Neurosurg. *55* (1981), 155—156.

161. Ljunggren, B., Brandt, L., Cronqvist, S., Kagström, E., Sundbärg, G., Säveland, H., Results of early surgery for ruptured intracranial aneurysms. Acta Neurochir. (Wien) *62* (1982), 112—113.

162. Loach, A. B., Benedict, C. R., Plasma catecholamine concentrations associated with cerebral vasospasms. J. Neurol. Sci. *45* (1980), 261—271.

163. Locksley, H. P., Report on the cooperative study of intracranial aneurysms and subarachnoid hemorrhage. J. Neurosurg. *25* (1966), 321—368.

164. Loew, F., Verbrauchskoagulopathie bei SAB? Dtsch. Med. Wochenschr. *101* (1976), 1472.

165. Loew, F., Wüstner, S., Diagnose, Behandlung und Prognose der traumatischen Hämatome des Schädelinneren. Acta Neurochir. (Wien) Suppl. *8* (1960), 1—158.

166. Van de Loo, J., Konservative Behandlung spontan aufgetretener intracerebraler Blutungen. In: Cerebrum, Blutgerinnung und Hämostase (Marx, R., Thies, H. A., Hrsg.), pp. 153—158. XXII. Hamburger Symposium über Blutgerinnung 1979. Wissenschaftlicher Dienst Roche 1980.

167. Mamoli, B., Sonneck, G., Lechner, K., Intrakranielle und spinale Blutungen bei Hämophilie. J. Neurol. *211* (1976), 143—154.

168. Markwardt, F., Therapie der Blutstillungsstörungen. Leipzig: J. A. Barth. 1972.
169. Markwardt, F. (Hrsg.), Fibrinolytics and antifibrinolytics. Handbuch der experimentellen Pharmakologie, Vol. 46. Berlin-Heidelberg-New York: Springer. 1978.
170. Markwardt, F., Diskussion in: Blutungen bei Kindern, Jugendlichen und Erwachsenen. In: Cerebrum, Blutgerinnung und Hämostase (Marx, R., Thies, H. A., Hrsg.), pp. 213—225. XXII. Hamburger Symposium über Blutgerinnung 1979. Wissenschaftlicher Dienst Roche 1980.
171. Markwardt, F., Zur Anwendung von Hämostyptica bei intrazerebralen Blutungen. In: Zerebrale Hypoxie und Ischämie vaskulär-zirkulatorischer Ätiologie (Schneider, D., Hrsg.), pp. 168—170, Diskussion: pp. 187—193. Leipzig: J. A. Barth. 1982.
172. Markwardt, F., Klöcking, H. P., Richter, M., Die Bestimmung synthetischer Antifibrinolytica in Körperflüssigkeiten und Organen. Pharmazie *22* (1967), 83—87.
173. Markwardt, F., Landmann, H., Klöcking, H. P., Fibrinolytika und Antifibrinolytika. Jena: G. Fischer. 1972.
174. Marx, R., Thies, H. A. (Hrsg.), Cerebrum, Blutgerinnung und Hämostase. XXII. Hamburger Symposium über Blutgerinnung 1979. Wissenschaftlicher Dienst Roche 1980.
175. Matis, P., Wirkungen von Trasylol auf Blutgerinnung und Wundheilung. Neue Aspekte der Trasylol Therapie, Vol. 2, pp. 19—38. Stuttgart-New York: F. K. Schattauer. 1968.
176. Matjasko, M., Ducker, T. B., Disseminated intravascular coagulation associated with removal of a primary brain tumor. Case report. J. Neurosurg. *47* (1977), 476—486.
177. Matsunaga, M., Yonemasu, Y., Takeda, S., Ohsato, K., Coagulation and fibrinolytic activities of the blood after subarachnoid hemorrhage. Blood and Vessel *9* (1978), 243—247. In Japanese.
178. Matsuo, O., Kato, K., Mihara, H., Okuno, S., Matsuo, T., Determination of α_2-Plasmin inhibitor in body fluids. Thromb. Res. *27* (1982), 555—562.
179. Maurice-Williams, R. S., Prolonged antifibrinolysis: An effective nonsurgical treatment for ruptured intracranial aneurysms? Brit. Med. J. *1* (1978), 945—947.
180. Maurice-Williams, R. S., Gordon, Y. B., Sykes, A., Monitoring fibrinolytic activity in the cerebrospinal fluid after aneurysmal subarachnoid haemorrhage—Guide to the risk of rebleeding? J. Neurol. Neurosurg. Psychiatry *43* (1980), 175—180.
181. Mendelow, A. D., Stockdill, G., Steers, A. J. W., Hayes, J., Gillingham, F. J., Double-blind trial of aspirin in patients receiving tranexamic acid for subarachnoid haemorrhage. Acta Neurochir. (Wien) *62* (1982), 195—202.
182. Merrem, B., Modellversuche zur Hämodynamik intrakranieller Aneurysmen. Zentralbl. Neurochir. *35* (1974), 35—49.
183. Mettinger, K. L., Egberg, N., A study of hemostasis in ischemic cerebrovascular disease. I.–III. Thromb. Res. *26* (1982), 183—210.
184. Mihara, H., Fujii, T., Okamoto, S., Fibrinolytic activity of cerebrospinal

fluid and the development of artificial cerebral haematomas in dogs. Thromb. Diath. Haemorrh. *21* (1969), 294—303.

185. Mihara, H., Tovi, D., Thulin, C. A., Fibrinolytic activity in experimental subarachnoid bleeding in dogs. Kobe J. Med. Sci. *19* (1973), 1—11.
186. Millikan, C. H., Cerebral vasospasm and ruptured intracranial aneurysm. Arch. Neurol. *32* (1975), 433—449.
187. Moltke, P., Investigations sur la teneur du système nerveux central en activateur de plasminogène. Tr. 6th Congress Eur. Soc. Haematol. *2* (1957), 475—477.
188. Mücke, R., Zur operativen Therapie von intrakraniellen Blutungen. In: Cerebrum, Blutgerinnung und Hämostase (Marx, R., Thies, H. A., Hrsg.). XXII. Hamburger Symposium über Blutgerinnung 1979. Wissenschaftlicher Dienst Roche 1980.
189. Mullan, S., Conservative management of the recently ruptured aneurysm. Surg. Neurol. *3* (1975), 27—32.
190. Mullan, S., Dawley, J., Antifibrinolytic therapy for intracranial aneurysms. J. Neurosurg. *28* (1968), 21—23.
191. Murano, G., The "Hageman" Connection: Interrelationships of blood coagulation, fibrino(geno)lysis, kinin generation and complement activation. Am. J. Hematol. *4* (1978), 409—417.
192. Murano, G., Bick, R. L. (eds.), Basic concepts of hemostasis and thrombosis. Boca Raton, Florida: CRC Press, Inc. 1980.
193. Nerke, O., Liquorzirkulationsstörungen. Fortschr. Neurol. Psychiatr. *44* (1976), 462—488.
194. Newman, R. L., A method for detecting and estimating plasminogen in cerebrospinal fluid. J. Clin. Pathol. *17* (1964), 313—315.
195. Nibbelink, D. W., Antifibrinolytic activity during administration of epsilon-aminocaproic acid. Stroke *2* (1971), 555—558.
196. Nibbelink, D. W., Cooperative aneurysm study: Antihypertensive and antifibrinolytic therapy following subarachnoid haemorrhage from ruptured intracranial aneurysms. In: Cerebral Vascular Diseases (Whisnant, J. P., Sandok, B. A., eds.), pp. 155—173. Ninth Princeton Conference. New York: Grune and Stratton 1975.
197. Nibbelink, D. W., Sahs, A. L., Antifibrinolytic therapy and drug-induced hypotension in treatment of ruptured intracranial aneurysms. (Preliminary report.) Trans. Am. Neurol. Assoc. *97* (1972), 145—152.
198. Nibbelink, D. W., Torner, J. C., Henderson, W. G., Intracranial aneurysms and subarachnoid hemorrhage. A cooperative study. Antifibrinolytic therapy in recent onset subarachnoid hemorrhage. Stroke *6* (1975), 622—629.
199. Nibbelink, D. W., Torner, J. C., Henderson, W. G., Intracranial aneurysms and subarachnoid hemorrhage—report on an randomized treatment study (4). A regulated bed rest. Stroke *8* (1977), 202—214.
200. Niewiarowski, S., Hausmanowa-Petrusewicz, I., Wegrzynowicz, Z., Blood clotting factors in cerebrospinal fluid. J. Clin. Pathol. *15* (1962), 497—500.
201. Nilsson, B. W., Cerebral blood flow in patients with subarachnoid haemorrhage studied with an intravenous isotope technique. Its clinical

significance in the timing of surgery of cerebral arterial aneurysm. Acta Neurochir. (Wien) *37* (1977), 33—48.
202. Norlen, G., Thulin, C. A., Experiences with epsilon-aminocaproic acid in neurosurgery. (A preliminary report.) Neurochirurgia (Stuttgart) *10* (1967), 81—86.
203. Norlen, G., Thulin, C. A., The use of antifibrinolytic substances in ruptured intracranial aneurysms. Neurochirurgia (Stuttgart) *12* (1969), 100—102.
204. Ohler, W., Blutstillungs- und Blutgerinnungsstörungen. Baden-Baden-Brüssel: Witzstrock. 1973.
205. Ohta, H., Ito, Z., Yasui, N., Suzuki, A., Extensive evacuation of subarachnoid clot for prevention of vasospasm—Effective or not? Acta Neurochir. (Wien) *63* (1982), 111—116.
206. Onoyama, K., Tahaka, K., Fibrinolytic activity of the arterial wall. Thromb. Diath. Haemorrh. *21* (1969), 1—11.
207. Pandolfi, M., Histochemistry and assay of plasminogen activator(s). Eur. J. Clin. Biol. Sci. *17* (1972), 254—260.
208. Park, B. E., Spontaneous subarachnoid hemorrhage complicated by communicating hydrocephalus: Epsilon-aminocaproic acid as a possible predisposing factor. Surg. Neurol. *11* (1979), 73—80.
209. Pasqualin, A., da Pian, R., An analysis of vasospasm following early surgery for intracranial aneurysms. Acta Neurochir. (Wien) *63* (1982), 153—159.
210. Patterson, R. H., Harpel, P., The effect of epsilon aminocaproic acid and tranexamic acid on thrombus size and strength in a simulated arterial aneurysm. J. Neurosurg. *34* (1971), 365—371.
211. Perlick, E., Bergmann, A., Gerinnungslaboratorium in Klinik und Praxis. Leipzig: G. Thieme. 1971.
212. Peterson, H. I., Peterson, A., Zederfeldt, B., Fibrinolytic activity in healing wound. Chir. Scand. *135* (1969), 649—652.
213. Pia, H. W., Langmaid, C., Zierski, J. (eds.), Cerebral Aneurysms. Advances in Diagnosis and Therapy. Berlin-Heidelberg-New York: Springer. 1979.
214. Pissarek, V., Analyse und Wertung der i.th. AFT mit PAMBA im Rahmen des konservativen Behandlungskonzepts der SAB. Eine klinische Studie. Erfurt. Medizinische Dissertation. 1981.
215. Porter, J. M., Acinapura, A. J., Kapp, J. P., Silver, D., Fibrinolytic activity of the spinal fluid and meninges. Surg. Forum *17* (1966), 425—427.
216. Porter, J. M., Acinapura, A. J., Kapp, J. P., Silver, D., Fibrinolysis in the central nervous system. Neurology (N.Y.) *19* (1969), 47—52.
217. Post, K. D., Flamm, E. S., Goodgold, A., Ransohoff, J., Ruptured intracranial aneurysms. Case morbidity and mortality. J. Neurosurg. *46* (1977), 290—295.
218. Profeta, G., Castellano, F., Guarnieri, L., Cigliano, A., Ambrosio, A., Antifibrinolytic therapy in the treatment of subarachnoid haemorrhage caused by arterial aneurysms. J. Neurosurg. Sci. (1975), 77—78.
219. Proud, G., Chamberlain, J., Anaphylactic reaction to aprotinin. (Letter) Lancet *II* (1976), 48—49.
220. Ramirez-Lassepas, M., Antifibrinolytic therapy in subarachnoid hemor-

rhage caused by ruptured intracranial aneurysm. Neurology (N.Y.) *31* (1981), 316—322.
221. Ransohoff, J., Goodgold, A., Benjamin, M. V., Pre-operative management of patients with ruptured intracranial aneurysms. J. Neurosurg. *36* (1972), 525—530.
222. Rapoport, S. T., Blood-brain in physiology and medicine. New York: Raven Press. 1976.
223. Raue, F., Die Gerinnung blutigen Liquors. Klin. Wochenschr. *4* (1925), 265—266.
224. Renkin, E. M., Transport of large molecules across capillary walls. Physiologist *7* (1964), 13—18.
225. Reuther, P., Fuhrmeister, U., Antifibrinolytic drugs in subarachnoid haemorrhage. Proceedings of the 33rd annual meeting. Acta Neurochir. (Wien) *62* (1982), 121.
226. Rieselbach, R. E., di Chiro, G., Freireich, E. J., Rall, D. P., Subarachnoid distribution of drugs after lumbar injection. N. Engl. J. Med. *267* (1962), 1273—1278.
227. Roach, M. R., Blood flow and thrombosis, particularly in aneurysms. Thromb. Diath. Haemorrh. Suppl. *59* (1974), 123—138.
228. Van Rossum, J., Wintzen, A. R., Endtz, L. J., Effect of tranexamic acid on rebleeding after subarachnoid hemorrhage: A double-blind controlled clinical trial. Ann. Neurol. *2* (1977), 242—245.
229. Rupprecht, A., Zur Differentialdiagnose des blutigen Liquors. Wien. Z. Nervenheilk. Suppl. *1* (1966), 113—115.
230. Russell, C. K., Spontaneous subarachnoid haemorrhage. Can. Med. Assoc. J. *28* (1933), 133—135.
231. Rydin, E., Lundberg, P. O., Tranexamic acid and intracranial thrombosis. (Letter) Lancet *II* (1976), 49.
232. Samama, M., Starkman, C., Horellou, M. H., Conard, J., Brami, R., Acar, J., Coagulation intravasculaire disséminée chronique dans un cas d'anévrysme ventriculaire. Arch. Mal. Coeur. *74* (1981), 111—116.
233. Sano, K., Saito, I., Indication and timing of operation and vasospasm. In: Cerebral Aneurysms. Advances in Diagnosis and Therapy (Pia, H. W., Langmaid, C., Zierski, J., eds.). Berlin-Heidelberg-New York: Springer. 1979.
234. Sartor, K., Spontanverschluß arteriovenöser Mißbildungen des Gehirns. Nervenarzt *49* (1978), 34—37.
235. Sasaki, T., Wakai, S., Asano, T., Takakura, K., Sano, K., Prevention of cerebral vasospasm after SAH with a thromboxane synthetase inhibitor, OKY-1581. J. Neurosurg. *57* (1982), 74—82.
236. Schaltenbrand, G., Allgemeine Neurologie, Pathophysiologie, klinische Untersuchungsmethoden, Syndrome. Stuttgart: G. Thieme. 1969.
237. Schemm, G. W., Blood clot adsorption and organization in the cerebrospinal fluid. Surg. Forum *17* (1966), 423—425.
238. Schemm, C., Bentley, J., Doerfler, M., Wound healing in the subarachnoid space. Neurology (N.Y.) *18* (1968), 862—869.

239. Schisano, G., The use of antifibrinolytic drugs in aneurysmal subarachnoid hemorrhage. Surg. Neurol. *10* (1978), 217—222.
240. Schmidt, R. M., Der Liquor cerebrospinalis. Untersuchungsmethodik und Diagnostik. Berlin: Volk und Gesundheit. 1968.
241. Schmidt-Matthiesen, H., Die fibrinolytische Aktivität von Endometrium und Myometrium, Dezidua und Plazenta, Kollum- und Korpuskarzinomen. Bibl. Gynaec. (Basel) *44* (1967), 1—117.
242. Schneck, S. A., von Kaulla, K. N., Fibrinolysis and the nervous system. Neurology (N.Y.) *11* (1961), 959—969.
243. Schuller, E., Lefevre, M., Tömpe, L., Electroimmunodiffusion of α_2M, IgA and IgG in nanogram quantities with a hydroxyethyl-cellulose-agarose gel: Application to unconcentrated CSF. Clin. Chim. Acta *42* (1972), 5—13.
244. Sedlarik, K., Blutgerinnung und Fibrinolyse bei der Wundheilung. Z. Aerztl. Fortb. (Jena) *71* (1977), 722—725.
245. Sengupta, R. P., So, S. C., Villarejo-Ortega, F. J., Use of epsilon aminocaproic acid (EACA) in the pre-operative management of ruptured intracranial aneurysms. J. Neurosurg. *44* (1976), 479—484.
246. Shapiro, S. S., Anderson, D. P., Thrombin inhibition in normal plasma. In: Chemistry and Biology of Thrombin (Lundblad, R. L., Fenton, J. W., Mann, K. G., eds.), pp. 361—374. Ann Arbor: Ann Arbor Sci. Publ. Inc. 1977.
247. Shaw, M. D. M., Miller, J. D., Epsilon-aminocaproic acid and subarachnoid haemorrhage. (Letter) Lancet *II* (1974), 847—848.
248. Shucart, W. A., Hussain, S. K., Cooper, P. R., Epsilon aminocaproic acid and recurrent subarachnoid hemorrhage. A clinical trial. J. Neurosurg. *53* (1980), 28—31.
249. Sicuteri, F., Treatment of subarachnoid and other intracranial hemorrhages with proteinase inhibitors. Ann. N.Y. Acad. Sci. (1971), 683—700.
250. Sicuteri, F., Fancuillacri, M., Bavazzaro, A., Frachi, G., del Branco, P. L., Kinins and intracranial hemorrhage. Angiology *21* (1970), 193—198.
251. Slade, W. R., Rabiner, A. M., Plasma thromboplastin antecedent deficiency and subarachnoid hemorrhage. Angiology *24* (1973), 533—537.
252. Smith, R. R., Upchurch, J. J., Monitoring antifibrinolytic therapy in subarachnoid hemorrhage. J. Neurosurg. *38* (1973), 339—344.
253. Sonntag, V. K. H., Stein, B. M., Arteriopathic complications during treatment of subarachnoid haemorrhage with epsilon-aminocaproic acid. J. Neurosurg. *40* (1974), 480—485.
254. Spallone, A., Antifibrinolytics in aneurysmal subarachnoid haemorrhage. A retrospective comparison of two different forms of antifibrinolytic therapy. Acta Neurochir. (Wien) *63* (1982), 245—250.
255. Stamm, H., Einführung in die Klinik der Fibrinolyse. Basel-New York: S. Karger. 1962.
256. Stoica, E., Cherciulescu, F., The dynamics of induced fibrinolysis in cerebrovascular accidents. Confin. neurol. (Basel) *27* (1966), 276—294.
257. Stürzebecher, J., Untersuchungen zur Reaktionsweise des Heparins. Folia Haematol. (Leipzig) *104* (1977), 731—739.
258. Suzuki, J. (ed.), Cerebral aneurysms. Tokyo: Neuron. 1979.

259. Suzuki, J., Onuma, T., Yoshimoto, T., Results of early operations on cerebral aneurysms. Surg. Neurol. *11* (1979), 407—412.
260. Suzuki, S., Sobata, E., Ando, A., Iwabuchi, T., Anaerobic change of bloody CSF in subarachnoid haemorrhage. Its relation to cerebral vasospasm. Acta Neurochir. (Wien) *58* (1981), 15—26.
261. Symon, L., Perspectives in aneurysm surgery. Acta Neurochir. (Wien) *63* (1982), 5—13.
262. Takashima, S., Koga, M., Tanaka, K., Fibrinolytic activity of human brain and cerebrospinal fluid. Brit. J. exp. Pathol. *50* (1969), 533—539.
263. Tanaka, M., Arch. Japan. Chir. *29* (1960), 449—453. In Japanese.
264. Tang, B. H., McKenna, P. J., Rovit, R. L., Primary fibrinolytic syndrome associated with subarachnoid hemorrhage. A case report. Angiology *24* (1973), 627—634.
265. Thies, H. A., Menschliche und tierische Gewebsthrombokinasen. Stuttgart: G. Thieme. 1957.
266. Toda, N., Ozaki, T., Ohta, T., Cerebrovascular sensitivity to vasoconstricting agents induced by subarachnoid hemorrhage and vasospasm in dogs. J. Neurosurg. *46* (1977), 296—303.
267. Todd, A. A., Nunn, A., Fibrinolytic activity in tissues and thrombi. In: Acta of the first international symposium on tissue factors in the homeostasis of the coagulation-fibrinolysis system. Florence: 1967, pp. 57—77.
268. Tovi, D., Studies on fibrinolysis in the central nervous system with special reference to intracranial haemorrhages and to the effect of antifibrinolytic drugs. Umea University Medical Dissertations No. 8. 1972.
269. Tovi, D., Fibrinolytic activity of human brain. A histochemical study. Acta Neurol. Scand. *49* (1973), 152—162.
270. Tovi, D., The use of antifibrinolytic drugs to prevent early recurrent aneurysmal subarachnoid haemorrhage. Acta Neurol. Scand. *49* (1973), 163—175.
271. Tovi, D., Preoperative management of patients with aneurysmal subarachnoid hemorrhage. J. Neurosurg. Sci. *19* (1975), 59—64.
272. Tovi, D., Nilsson, I. M., Increased fibrinolytic activity and fibrin degradation products after experimental intracerebral haemorrhage. Acta Neurol. Scand. *48* (1972), 403—415.
273. Tovi, D., Nilsson, I. M., Thulin, C. A., Fibrinolysis and subarachnoid haemorrhage. Inhibitory effect of tranexamic acid. A clinical study. Acta Neurol. Scand. *48* (1972), 393—402.
274. Tovi, D., Nilsson, I. M., Thulin, C. A., Fibrinolytic activity of the cerebrospinal fluid after subarachnoid haemorrhage. Acta Neurol. Scand. *49* (1973), 1—9.
275. Tovi, D., Thulin, C. A., Ability of tranexamic acid to cross the blood-brain barrier and its use in patients with ruptured intracranial aneurysms. Acta Neurol. Scand. *48* (1972), 257.
276. Towart, R., The pathophysiology of cerebral vasospasm, and pharmacological approaches to its management. Acta Neurochir. (Wien) *63* (1982), 253—258.
277. Tubbs, R. R., Benjamin, S. P., Dohn, D. E., Recurrent subarachnoid

hemorrhage associated with aminocaproic acid therapy and acute renal artery thrombosis. Case report. J. Neurosurg. *51* (1979), 94—97.
278. Tzonos, T., Runa, B., Die Wirkung von Proteinasen und Fibrinolyseinhibitoren auf das experimentelle Hirnoedem. Z. Neurol. *205* (1973), 61—70.
279. Uttley, A. H. C., Buckell, M., Biochemical changes after spontaneous subarachnoid haemorrhage. III. Coagulation and lysis with special reference to recurrent haemorrhage. J. Neurol. Neurosurg. Psychiatry *31* (1968), 621—627.
280. Uttley, D., Richardson, A. E., ε-aminocaproic acid and subarachnoid haemorrhage. (Letter) Lancet *II* (1974), 1080—1081.
281. Vahar-Matiar, H., Müller, H. J., Lippes, G., Der blutige Liquor. Acta Neurochir. (Wien) *29* (1973), 229—245.
282. Vermeulen, M., van Gijn, J., Hijdra, A., Concerning the paper written by Adams, H. P., *et al.*: Antifibrinolytic therapy in patients with aneurysmal subarachnoid hemorrhage. Adams, H. P., Sahs, A. L., Torner, J.: Reply to the letter of Vermeulen, M., *et al.* Arch. *39* (1982), 384.
283. Vermeulen, M., Muizelaar, J. P., Do antifibrinolytic agents prevent rebleeding after rupture of a cerebral aneurysm? A review. Clin. Neurol. Neurosurg. *82* (1980), 25—30.
284. Vermylen, J. G., Chamone, D. A. F., The role of the fibrinolytic system in thromboembolism. Prog. Cardiovasc. Dis. *21* (1979), 255—266.
285. Vilchez, J. J., Aznar, J. A., Benedito, J., Tascon, A., Conzales, A., Jimenez, C., Vilela, C., Fibrinólisis local en hemorragias cerebrales y subaracnoideas. Rev. Clin. Esp. *150* (1978), 193—195.
286. Vivenza, C., Pian, R. D. A., The use of antifibrinolytic drugs in the management of subarachnoid hemorrhage due to aneurysmal rupture. Acta Neurochir. (Wien) *48* (1979), 131.
287. De Vivo, D., Kline, E., Dodge, P. R., Influence of human cerebrospinal fluid on blood coagulation. Arch. Neurol. *13* (1965), 615—620.
288. Walter, W., Schiefek, W., Zur Klinik und Prognose der Subarachnoidealblutung ohne angiographischen Nachweis einer Gefäßmißbildung. Med. Welt *20* (1969), 1600—1608.
289. Watanabe, H., Ishii, S., Matsuda, T., Studies on the fibrinolytic system in ruptured intracranial aneurysm. Neurol. Surg. No shinkei Geka (Japan) *6* (1978), 563—569.
290. Watanabe, H., Ito, M., Chigasaki, H., Ishii, S., Antifibrinolytic therapy in ruptured intracranial aneurysm through repeated monitoring of fibrinolytic activity of blood. Neurol. Med. Chir. (Tokyo) *16* (1980), 91—96.
291. Werner, A., Sofortoperationen nach SAB? Dtsch. Med. Wochenschr. *105* (1976), 3—4.
292. Wieczorek, V., Brodkorb, W., Remde, W., Subarachnoidalblutung bei verstärkter Fibrinolyse. Münch. Med. Wochenschr. *112* (1970), 366—369.
293. Wiegershausen, B., Riethling, A. K., Paegelow, I., Reichel, A., Einige pharmakologische Aspekte zur Mikrozirkulation und Permeation. In: Gefäßwand und Blutplasma IV (Emmrich, R., Hrsg.), pp. 151—157. Jena: G. Fischer. 1974.

294. Wilkins, R. H., Smith, W., Anlyan, W. G., Hetherington, D. C., Woodhall, B., The effect of normal cerebrospinal fluid on blood clotting and fibroblast growth. J. Surg. Res. *1* (1961), 260—265.
295. Wiman, B., Boman, L., Collen, D., On the kinetics of the reaction between human antiplasmin and a low-molecular-weight form of plasmin. Eur. J. Biochem. *87* (1978), 143—146.
296. Wiman, B., Collen, D., Molecular mechanism of physiological fibrinolysis. Nature *272* (1978), 549—550.
297. Wintzen, A. R., van Rossum, J., ε-aminocaproic acid in prevention of subarachnoid haemorrhage. Lancet *8125* (1979), 1084—1085.
298. Wu, K. Y., Jacobsen, C. D., Hoak, J. C., Plasminogen in human and abnormal human cerebrospinal fluid. Arch. Neurol. *28* (1973), 64—66.
299. Yamaura, A., Nakamura, T., Makino, H., Hagihara, Y., Cerebral complication of antifibrinolytic therapy in the treatment of ruptured intracranial aneurysm. Animal experiment and a review of literature. Eur. Neurol. *19* (1980), 77—87.
300. Yaşargil, M. G., Yonekawa, Y., Zumstein, B., Stahl, H. G., Hydrocephalus following spontaneous subarachnoid haemorrhage, clinical features and treatment. J. Neurosurg. *39* (1973), 474—479.
301. Yours, S., Farina, M. L., Levati, A., Paino, R., Myocardial infarction during antifibrinolytic treatment of subarachnoid haemorrhage. Thromb. Haemost. *42* (1979), 1347—1348.
302. Zetter, B. R., Gospodarowicz, D., The effect of thrombin on endothelial cell proliferation. In: Chemistry and Biology of Thrombin (Lundblad, R. L., Fenton, J. W., Mann, K. G., eds.), pp. 551—558. Ann Arbor: Ann Arbor Sci. Publ. Inc. 1977.
303. Cyclocapron-Tranexamsäure. Werbeschrift AB Kabi, Kabi Arzneimittel. Stockholm 1976.
304. Deutsches Arzneibuch, 7. Auflage, Diagnostische Laboratoriumsmethoden. Berlin: Akademie. 1968/1973.
305. Test-Fibel. Blutgerinnung, Klinik und Labor. Mannheim: Boehringer Biochemica. 1973/1977.

